HEALING THREADS

About the author

Mary Beith is a writer, lecturer and journalist, contributing articles on archaeology, folklore, traditional medicines and current Highland issues to newspapers and magazines. She lives in Sutherland, in the north of Scotland.

HEALING THREADS

*Traditional Medicines
of the Highlands and Islands*

Mary Beith

Birlinn

For my father and Paddy

This edition published in 2004 by
Birlinn Limited
West Newington House
10 Newington Road
Edinburgh
EH9 1QS

www.birlinn.co.uk

First published in 1995 by Polygon, Edinburgh

ISBN 1 84158 277 8

British Library Cataloguing-in-Publication Data
A catalogue record for this book is available
from the British Library

Printed and bound by Creative Print & Design, Wales

CONTENTS

PREFACE AND ACKNOWLEDGEMENTS

This book might more accurately, if less invitingly, be called 'A Taste of Highland Medicine', since all the details of the subject would fill several volumes. Some may find the initial accent on Celtic art and metaphysics at odds with a systematic approach. Those of more 'mystical' inclinations may balk at attempts to find a rational basis for enigmatic rituals. But the healers themselves blended common sense and the supernatural – to understand and do justice to their approach to medicine, we must meet them half way.

I was touched by George Henderson's remark (page 102) on a treatment for epilepsy: 'my thoughts were at the heart of things'. If we aim at that 'heart' we may begin to grasp the theory behind the practice. Pre-industrial societies believed in the remedial use of drama, and I am interested in exploring how the intellect behind Celtic arts is reflected in the philosophy of healing.

Many people gave advice, information and support and I am grateful to each and every one of them. Above all, I want to thank Ronald Black, who introduced me to the medieval Gaelic medical works and urged the writing of this book. Ronnie has been a constant, expert and patient source of insight and encouragement, and assiduous in checking manuscript and proofs. Many, many, thanks, too, to Máire Black, who, as well as helping in other ways, encouraged me to attempt a bit more than just a book of facts.

Special thanks also to Ian McCormack and the *West Highland Free*

Press for publishing my column on traditional medicines, and Donald Omand and Donald Paterson of Aberdeen University, for arranging lectures (the articles and talks have brought links with a diversity of people with interesting tales and knowledge); and to Allan Macinnes, Trevor Cowie, Alan Saville and Malcolm Nicolson for reading the manuscript and making expert comments. All errors of interpretation or fact, needless to say, are mine, and I am happy to provoke debate, and invite ideas, information and criticism.

A generous grant from the Sir John Macdonald Study Fund enabled far wider inquiries than might have been possible, and I am much indebted to the faith shown by Rob Macdonald Parker and the Clan Donald Trust. I am also grateful to Mrs Dixie Miller and the Northern Studies Centre for helping to fund a trip to Leiden.

And now for the hardest bit, for it is impossible to name each contributor of information or encouragement. But I am particularly grateful to the following, either for constant help or for random inspired remarks or details which helped so much else fall into place: Robert Anderson, Owen Beith, Margaret Bennett, David Caldwell, Michael Carmichael, Hugh Cheape, Isobel Cross, Julia Cross, Andrew Currie, Barbara Fairweather, Valerie and William Gillies, John Holliday, David Hamilton, Fiona Howard, Malcolm Ingram, Jacqueline Jenkinson, Jim Johnston, Malcolm Bangor Jones, Terry Keatinge, the late Kirsty Larner, Hazel Lindsay, Patrick Logan, Antonie Luyendijk, Donald Meek, Mairi MacArthur, Janet and Alfred McClintock, Archie Macdonald, Chrissie Macdonald, Hugh Macdonald, Janet Macdonald, Joan Macdonald, Ann MacDonell, Mary McGinley, the late Andrew Mackay, Joseph Mackay, Margaret Mackay, Betty Mackenzie, Tom Mackenzie, Donald Angie Maclean, Sorley Maclean, Agnes Maclennan, Robert Maclennan, Finlay Macleod, Flora and Hector Macphail, Donald MacRurie, Colin Michie, Roger Miket, Brian Moffat, Mary Montgomery, Jimmy and Jean Morrison, Ruth and Stuart Nairn, John Purser, Anna and Graham Ritchie, Chris Robinson, Mairead Ross, Margaret Fay Shaw, Sandy

Sutherland, Frank Thompson and Caroline Wickham-Jones. A big thank you, too, to those who wished to remain anonymous but gave some very valuable insights.

Special mention among library and archive sources must go to the School of Scottish Studies and the Royal Pharmaceutical Society; to Margaret Coutts, first of Glasgow University Library and now of the Queen Mother Library, Aberdeen; Penny Collett and Norman Newton, Inverness public library; Olive Geddes, National Library of Scotland; Mère Marie Madeleine, Abbaye de Ste Cecile, Solesmes; Pat and Elliot Rudie, Strathnaver Museum; and Alistair Sinclair on the North West Sutherland mobile library van.

The skill and unstinting help of computer expert David Holmes restored the word-processor (and myself) to good tune during some very sticky moments. He cannot be thanked enough.

To my publisher Marion Sinclair and her friendly and efficient team at Polygon go my deep thanks for giving *Healing Threads* a smooth and untroubled birth.

No words are sufficient for the many great kindnesses shown by family, friends, neighbours and local businesses during my prolonged pottering on this book. My thanks to them are boundless.

. . . .

Thanks for permission to quote: to John Bannerman for an extract from *The Beatons*; Carcanet Press, for lines from C.H. Sisson's *In a Trojan Ditch*; Trevor Cowie, from *Magic Metal: Early Metalworkers in the North-East*; Faber & Faber, for extracts from P.V. Glob's *The Mound People*; Barbara Fairweather, *Highland Plant Lore*; Anna Ritchie and the Society of Antiquaries of Scotland for extracts from 'Painted pebbles in early Scotland', in *PSAS*, 104; and Derick Thomson for permission to use material from *An Introduction to Gaelic Poetry* and from 'Gaelic Learned Orders and Literati in Medieval Scotland', in *Scottish Studies*, vol. 12. All quotations from these and other known origins are fully acknowledged either in the main text or in the source notes.

INTRODUCTION

AMBIGUITIES OF ART AND HEALING

Many writers on the Highlands and islands of Scotland have given tantalising glimpses of a local healing tradition that combines common sense and mysticism in a vigorous blend. Yet there has been a curious neglect of a wide view of the whole body of that tradition. My aim in writing *Healing Threads* is to fill that gap by giving a general historical background as well as describing an extensive, though not exhaustive, variety of remedies. In this way, I hope to show how a concept of healing, by virtue of its survival from ancient times until quite recently, may help to shed further light on a Celtic perspective on life which once pervaded the whole British Isles and much of mainland Europe.

The roots of folk medicine are diffuse and partly lie in a succession of outdated or discarded official medical practices which reflect the attitudes and ideologies of their time and which in turn ultimately derive from the earliest folk remedies. In Britain it was only in 1858 that formal degrees in medicine were required before people could practice legally. Until then it was not unknown for practitioners to move casually between the two sectors. In less obvious ways, this long term interaction of folk and official medicine continues to the present day.

Gaelic traditional medicine has a strong association with the official Highland physicians of the middle ages. It also displays distinctly Celtic influences.

From medieval vernacular literature and oral traditions it is clear that the Celts had a talent for riddles and word-games. Classical authors, such as Lucan, Diodorus Siculus and Julius Caesar, tell how Celtic religion hinged on a belief in the transmigration of souls. Celtic art still teases the viewer with its intricacies and ambiguities, with abstract designs which transmute, in the eyes of the beholder, into human and animal shapes and seem to say: nothing is quite what it seems.

As with the legends, religion and art, Celtic medicine is a testimony to an intelligent observation of nature and an astute understanding of the weave of the human mind. If, politically, the Celts had no centre to hold them together, culturally a central strength radiates and pervades a range of themes. In a curious way it appears that even the configurations of their art are mirrored in the 'patterns' of healing incantations.

The strong Scottish, Irish and Welsh medical traditions that survived even into the early years of the twentieth century, had their foundation in a Celtic society which, in turn, had absorbed and refined the traditions of even earlier peoples.

I have called this book *Healing Threads* not so much because the use of threads in healing rituals was a peculiarly Gaelic or even Celtic practice, but more as an allusion to the unbroken cords linking the Celtic world with other cultures. Just as the Celts drew inspiration for art, religion and oral literature from many quarters and made the end-result unmistakably their own so, too, their medical traditions were linked to diverse sources and, in turn, their knowledge of the healing arts spread among other peoples. For example, in his *Natural History* (*c*.AD 78) the Roman writer, Pliny the Elder, reveals his fascination with the remedies of the Gauls, while the collection of medieval Gaelic medical manuscripts held in the National Library of Scotland contains numerous references to Greek and Arabic sources.

A sense of 'healing threads' permeates the understanding of the medical traditions of the Highlands and islands of Scotland, and Gaelic medicine is deeply interwoven into the story of the Gael as a whole. In describing this subject there is a need to be wary of a Highland backcloth that has lent itself only too often to a sentimentality and whimsy that can have one floundering in clichés. While there is nothing to be tritely sentimental about in the ravages of whooping cough, or boils and piles, the 'ancient wisdom' aspect remains a snare.

Just as the intricacies of Celtic art[1] are finely crafted, geometrically clever, and technically deft, something elusive remains, as if inviting a game between beholder and object. Abstract motifs trick us into a shape-shifting mood and the mind is diverted to an interplay both humorous and mystical. So in the medicine, a noticeable humour and a certain mysticism intertwine with practical knowledge and skill. A keen awareness of that humour is also vital to the researcher, not in order to derive some facile amusement from some of the stranger-seeming cures and rituals – but to prevent the modern mind from slipping into nostalgic banalities or from being too rigidly encased in its own prejudices.

It is also important to bear in mind that no human society is perfect, that there was no Golden Age of mystic knowledge, only a succession of varyingly tarnished ages whose 'esoteric wisdom' owed much to professional secrecy, self-preservation and expediency. Not a lot changes in the wider human conduct of affairs, and a strong healing tradition can have emerged only from the fact that a variety of ills needed treating. Nevertheless, it is beyond question that the medieval Gaels in particular had a basic belief in preventive medicine and the importance of maintaining health through diet, exercise and hygiene.

A dedicated handful of Victorian and early twentieth century pharmacists and physicians, who might have been expected to take a sceptical view of traditional Highland cures, showed a commendable lack of professional bias in their serious investigations of the subject in the not always sympathetic climate of the nineteenth century with its dismissal of 'old wives' tales'. Among them was the Kingussie-based chemist Alexander McCutcheon (1875–1927) whose analytical interest in local cures resulted in a thoughtful report to the North British Pharmaceutical Society: '[The] pharmacy of today is an advanced science, but we are working upon a heritage which has been calcined and refined in the crucible of experience.'[2]

For the most part, however, while there was an interest in folklore and much valuable work was done, the end result was only too often the recounting of practices as quaint and fossilised relics of the past, an entertaining museum of the human psyche. Unlike McCutcheon, few saw a contemporary orthodox relevance in rural remedies.

Out in the jungles of the Empire, the practices of tribal shamans were accorded even less respect by European explorers, but among those who took a deeper interest in indigenous ways of life, the inquiries in Africa of the Scots missionary doctor David Livingstone are particularly relevant. More recent biographies have shown the Victorian hero with a heart as well as feet of clay, a man who alienated his family, most of his companions, friends and fellow explorers with his selfishness and treated native African expedition helpers like mere slaves. But there is a lesser known side to Livingstone that links him in practice as well as by name and bloodline to the ancient traditions of Gaelic medicine.

At best, most European missionaries' attitudes to native traditions displayed a patronising tolerance and curiosity. Yet, whatever his perspectives and shortcomings in other directions, Livingstone stood apart from his colleagues in his views on native medicine. He not only closely questioned the Central African *sing'anga*, who were herbalists and healers rather than 'smellers-out of witches', on their philosophy, but he collected the roots and leaves they used in the hope of organising a materia medica. He was also keen for his British colleagues to respect local ways.

In 1858 he wrote to Dr John Kirk, medical officer to the Zambezi Expedition:

One especial means of gaining their favour will be by giving them the benefit of your medical skill and remedial air. They possess medical men among themselves who are generally the most observant people to be met with; it is desirable to be at all times on good terms with them . . . Slight complaints, except among the very poor, ought to be referred to their care, and severe cases, before being undertaken, should be enquired with the doctor himself and no disparaging remark ever made on the previous treatment in the presence of the patient. This line of conduct will lead to the more urgent cases only being referred to you; time and medicine will both be saved, while your influence will be extended.[3]

In this respect Livingstone's thinking and practice was 'radically different from most other missionaries and certainly very different from the majority of Europeans in Africa throughout most of the 20th century, let alone the 19th'.[4]

A clue to that difference may lie in the values passed down by Livingstone's ancestors. Gaelic medicine was in his blood. A direct descendant of the Mac Dhuinnshléibhe medical kindred – his grandfather came from the island of Ulva near Mull – he was heir to a unique inheritance that combined the scholarship of medieval Europe and the Near East with ancient folk traditions, and which had survived, if in increasingly diluted form, into the Highlands of his own time.

Where the attitude of his colleagues could be condescending when not highly arrogant, Livingstone approached the knowledge of the *sing'anga* in a genuine spirit of inquiry. At the same time, his own ancestors' knowledge, ironically, was being viewed as quaintly folksy by English and Lowland travellers from Boswell and Johnson onwards. Some, such as Allan Fullarton and Charles Baird who reported in 1838 that the Barra people 'pass from the cradle to the grave, in a state of ignorance as profound as that which characterises the New Zealander [i.e. the Maori native]', were downright dismissive of local culture. Unschooled as the Hebrideans may have been in the English language, and materially impoverished as they undoubtedly were, the particularly rich traditions of Barra and the language in which they had passed orally from generation to generation, were lost on the monoglot visitor. Notable, too, was the easy dismissal of the Maori tradition by 'civilised' Europeans whose own simmering tribalism was, under the war-mask of political philosophy, to erupt into the devastating bloodshed of the twentieth century. Seeing their own intrepid ventures into the 'remote' Highlands on a par with equally prejudiced treks into deepest Africa or the furthest Antipodes, such people simply reinforced their own ethnocentrism.[5]

The few who looked more seriously into the medical lore of the Gaels were impressed with the range and depth of knowledge of local healers and their far-reaching history. Towards the end of the nineteenth century, the Caledonian Medical Society[6] – founded in 1878 as a society for Highland medical students at Edinburgh and re-established in 1881 with a membership open to medical graduates of Highland descent – began to collect what remained of the knowledge of the methods and materia medica. The project was to develop from its beginnings in casual curiosity to a deeper professional regard for the old ways, and suggestions that there might be much of value to modern medicine.

Alas, the move fizzled out and today the papers read to the Society all those years ago, and especially the early volumes (1890–1910) which are rich in Highland healing lore, remain largely unknown to the general public. This neglect is in sharp contrast to the way in which, prompted mainly by the good work of the World Health Organisation, the traditional medicines of other countries, especially those of the Third World, have acquired a new lease of life.

Even less well known than the body of traditional cures is the great legacy of the medieval Gaelic medical manuscripts. Just as the clans had their *seanachaidhean*, the recognised and respected keepers of ancestral lore, who committed to memory clan sagas and genealogies, so, too, clans had their recognised healers and from the early fourteenth to the late seventeenth centuries these physicians collected and created a considerable body of scientific and learned literature.[7]

The bulk of the early Gaelic manuscripts in the National Library of Scotland consists of medical works dating from before 1700 when, despite the popular image of the 'wild' Gael, clan chiefs extended a valuable patronage to their doctors and other learned orders. While in number these make up only twenty-nine of the library's eighty-three Gaelic manuscripts from pre-eighteenth century Scotland, many are lengthy, some running to several hundred pages. These works belong to a tradition held in common by the professional Gaelic medical men of both Ireland and Scotland.[8] Not many of their texts have been edited and translated in full, but one which has, from a manuscript in the British Library, is the *Regimen Sanitatis*, or Rule of Health, of the Beatons – one of the more influential of the hereditary families of doctors – and its publication (in 1910) has had a limited circulation.

Many books on the Highlands and islands of Scotland have referred to the folk cures of the area. According to the quality of the work in question these have varied from a few examples of 'quaint' practices to a rather more respectful acknowledgement of the medical lore of the past.

Some works, such as Martin Martin's *A Description of the Western Islands of Scotland* (1703; rev. 1716) and Alexander Carmichael's *Carmina Gadelica* (six volumes, 1900–71), both containing an abundance of old remedies, are not as widely known as they deserve to be outside Scotland. Martin's reports were made at the behest of Robert Sibbald, appointed the first Professor of Medicine in Edinburgh in 1685, and it is likely that the outlook and practices of the then 'remote' Gael played a role in influencing the development of a world-famous centre for the practice and teaching of clinical medicine.

In his valuable work *The Beatons* (1986), John Bannerman diligently traces the background, education and family connections of one of the more widespread hereditary medical dynasties, so in this book I shall simply try to give a short account of their history and concentrate more on their remedies and the place they held in the esteem and memories of the people.

Highland healing should be set in the wider context of medieval European orthodox medicine so that the local use of, say, skulls, spiders, woodlice and snakes is seen as no more strange – even considerably less so – than the prescribing of powdered Egyptian mummy across seventeenth-century urban apothecaries' counters. Modern medicine, too, uses material derived from animal sources that would seem equally bizarre were they not served up in the form of white powders and odourless liquids and further sanitised with Latin names. There are also many instances where the old Highland practices have distinct counterparts with traditional medicines and methods throughout the world.

The 'healing threads' cross time as well as space. The ancient serpent 'helix' symbol of healing and communication, the spirals of Celtic art and the patterns arising from modern genetic research arrive in their different ways at a very similar visual perception of the enigma of life. On a more practical level, a nineteenth-century Cromarty woman who cut the liver from a mouse to treat a desperately ill child – who went on to make a full recovery – was echoing a practice known to the people of pre-dynastic Egypt in c.4000 BC. Today mice are used in laboratories for testing medicines or as a medium for the culture of antibodies – whether they will ever again become part of the materia medica itself is not necessarily an idle question. In today's rather more sensitive climate, investigations would be more likely to hinge on a chemical formula to be isolated from whatever it was that gave the humble mouse such long-lasting importance in the medicine of the ancients. In the Highlands, the genuine practice of folk medicine – that is to say, through necessity rather than whim – lingered on far longer than elsewhere in the British Isles, both geography and history having combined – 'conspired' may be as apt – to leave the area relatively isolated. A consequence was that between the demise of the clan physicians around the end of the seventeenth century and the introduction of the Government's Highlands & Islands Medical Scheme in 1919 good-quality professional medical care rarely penetrated the more remote areas.

A strong respect for tradition and the memories of the prestige of the clan medical system as well as an intelligent use of the materia medica and methods, reliance on common sense and a gifted psychological insight gave the Gaelic healers a solid base. Rituals, for example, often show an understanding of the use of drama and intensity of experience in healing by focusing the patient's mind and creating a significant psychological moment or impression.

What the Gaels also retained was a curious blend of innocence with their ancient knowledge. As will be seen in Chapters 6 and 13, practices which came to viewed by many ordinary citizens as well as the legislature and the churches as 'black and satanic' in other areas of Scotland and beyond, especially with regard to ritual and incantations, were seen in an altogether different context by the Gaels. Closer in spirit to the original motivation behind such practices, they saw beauty and purpose where others saw darkness and folly. This is not to say that old practices were not prey to corruption once divorced from their roots, nor that some Highland charmers or their clients were themselves immune to malice, but that in looking closely into the Gaelic healing tradition, many customs that came to be seen and practised as occult elsewhere begin to fall into place.

Much of Highland folklore has been seen and presented in a mood of nostalgia for a fairy otherworld, while much of the wider Scottish folklore has been presented with a darker side of witches and demons. In this book there is an attempt to strike a balance by simply looking at a practical – sometimes fallible, sometimes successful, always caring – human tradition of healing which embraced spiritual and mental as well as physical needs.

The book is arranged in two parts, the first giving the historical background and the second giving practical examples of the cures. Since it is intended as a general introduction to the traditional medicines of the Highlands and islands, I have not attempted to give a comprehensive account of every remedy or the variations practised in different districts. I have tried, however, to offer readers not only the overall picture but also to provide them with an insight into the outlook on life that characterised the Gaelic approach to healing.

The Gaelic pharmacy was a rich one whose sources lay almost entirely in nature and were usually subject to the minimum of preparation. While many materials are common to other folk traditions, the Gaels tended more towards 'simples' – i.e. the use of one herb at a time as a specific for a given ill. I am preparing a more extensive and fully annotated list of the materia medica and a copy will be lodged at the Clan Donald Centre, Armadale, Isle of Skye.

CAUTION: Many of the old remedies are quite innocuous and may even be useful but self-diagnosis can also be a self-deceptive activity; some of the herbs mentioned are poisonous, and others can have side-effects. In general it is an offence to uproot any wild plant without the landowner's permission and the rarest species are protected against all forms of collecting (including leaves, berries, etc). Excessive gathering of even very common flowers can cause damage or spoil the countryside for others.

HISTORY

1

ORIGINS

The world is divided.
There are two destinies:
a destiny for happiness
and the Devil's destiny.[1]

When Lachlann mac Thearlaich Òig, the seventeenth-century Gaelic poet, reputed to have inscribed the above words in his second wife's bible, was alive and perhaps happy in the parish of Strath in Skye, the destiny of Neil Beaton of Husabost in the same island was open to speculation.

On the one hand people would travel from as far as the Outer Isles or mainland Ross-shire to seek cures from the famous empiric. On the other, there were those who, as Martin Martin reported, suspected that Beaton's success 'proceeded rather from a Compact with the Devil, than from the Virtue of Simples'.

Although, on the whole, the Highlands were to be scarcely affected by the witchcraft persecutions of the sixteenth and seventeenth centuries (see Chapter 6), practitioners of traditional medicine could still be a target both of disgruntled neighbours and those who affected the 'advanced' attitudes of the south of Scotland and England. That the orthodox medicine of the period, involving as it did exotic preparations and 'scientific' latinised jargon, could be as arcane as folk healing, was ignored. In many ways the official medicine was even more ripe for suspicion, but the orthodox practitioners and apothecaries were a powerful body. Folk healers were largely poor, insecure and isolated.

Nevertheless, in Gaelic society they had the advantage of a long tradition of practice and knowledge that was still an essential part of a respected ancient culture vital to the Gaels' strong sense of identity. Such opprobrium as a few individuals met with seems mainly to have been in the general run of local squabbles and jealousies.

But where do the roots of that tradition start? The simplest, though necessarily vague, answer is when the first remedy effectively healed a wound, a disease or even just a sense of physical discomfort. Whenever and wherever it began it became, like medicine throughout the ancient world, inextricably involved with religion and ritual.

If the 'two destinies' could be split so starkly by religion into good and evil, similar concepts were also rooted deep in medical philosophy, with the difference that healing lay in the *balance* rather than the *conflict* of opposites. The enduring medical emblem of the caduceus – the snakes entwining Mercury's wand – which is still used by, for instance, the British Medical Association, symbolises this belief in interaction and renewal. Had it not had the sanction of a powerful lobby it might, in the late Middle Ages, have itself been taken for the very sign of the devil, for healing has always involved a sense of the mysterious.

Perhaps the earliest known depiction of a caduceus in a medical context is the one shown on a Sumerian goblet of the third millennium BC. Gaelic healing must rely on oral tradition rather than artefacts for its ancient provenance and it, too, has a story illustrating the importance of snake symbolism in medicine.[2] The story (given in Chapter 4) has been handed down in a medieval setting, but it bears all the signs of being an apocryphal one of much earlier origins.

Perhaps there was always a sense of 'two destinies' about medicine – life or death, cure or blunder, health or sickness. The responsibility was always enormous, with the need for the healer to be seen, in pagan or in monotheistic cultures, to be on the side of the gods with the rider that one man's god can be another man's demon. It is in societies deeply imbued with a suspicion that the search for the light of knowledge – as opposed to that of wisdom or understanding – brings the inquirer in touch with the powers of darkness, as in the Judaeo-Christian tradition, that there seems to be the strongest sense of those 'two destinies'. Each age has developed its own peculiar scruples. For some thirteen centuries from the time of Galen (AD 130–200) there was little advance in western European medicine, in contrast with, say, Arabian experimentalism, because the Church decreed that disease was the will of God. Today there are ethical debates about genetic research.

It is impossible to say whether the prehistoric mind worked along similar lines, but for this: the great wealth of knowledge about diseased states of mind and body, and the cures derived from a huge variety of sources, which emerge into the earliest written records. These can have had their source only in unchronicled centuries, indeed millennia, of positive inquiry, experimentation and learning handed down orally from generation to generation. The Gaels carried on that ancient tradition for, arguably, longer than any other western European society. Equally, only guesses can be made about the medical practices of prehistory.

Informed archaeological opinion based on evidence from known early skeletons has it that, on the whole, most people died at or before what we would now consider middle age. It is not unusual to find prehistoric skeletons with signs of arthritis and osteoporosis which may or may not have been treated and people who had suffered broken bones and violent deaths. Ancient burials also indicate the status of the individual and often yield valuable information on how society functioned as well as its perceptions of death and a possible afterlife. Although a large-scale survey and analysis of pre-medieval skeletons has yet to be undertaken in Scotland and evidence remains patchy, there are some interesting differences between medieval and prehistoric skeletons. For example, Bronze Age skeletons have shown that people then were a great deal taller (and tall even in modern terms) than the inhabitants of medieval burghs, revealing that a healthier diet and way of life enabled prehistoric people to reach their growth potential. However, the majority of medieval bones come from the cemeteries and unmarked graves of common people and, in all likelihood, the Bronze Age skeletons are representative only of a ruling élite. Experts look forward to the time, perhaps not too far away, when funding will become available to conduct a wide-ranging survey of prehistoric human remains in Scotland. Until such time it is impossible to gain a proper picture either of how those societies functioned or what general standards of health pertained.

Soil samples taken by archaeologists can now reveal a lot by way of pollen analysis but it is usually impossible to say, especially in prehistoric contexts, which of the plants indicated were used for floor coverings, bedding, brewing or food, and which for medicinal purposes, and a number of the species may simply have occurred incidentally.

However, so many shrivelled outer skins of a type of puffball mushroom were found in the 1970s at the 5000 year old Neolithic village of Skara Brae in Orkney that archaeologists could agree only that the inhabitants must have had a purpose for them. These skins, it has been agreed, were a rare piece of evidence that pointed to a herbal medicine.

They may have had many uses. Where the whole puffball provides a useful and tasty food when it is young, traditional medicine only makes use of the insides of the mature fungus, hence the assumption that the Skara Brae puffballs were used in healing. The inner tissue makes a handy, and effective, styptic for cuts and wounds; and the spores may be used – with skill and caution – as a form of anaesthetic. In the old days country people also used the smoke from burning puffballs to stupefy wild bees so that honey could be gathered with impunity. (For information on the use of herbs and other materia medica see Part II.)

Today there is a strong tendency to view Orcadians as the inheritors of a predominantly Norse culture but there is no denying them an earlier Celtic Iron Age heritage and, before then, a culturally linked – in broad terms, at least – prehistory with the areas which were later to become Gaelic-speaking. The puffballs of Skara Brae would have been no isolated experiment and it is reasonable to view them as the earliest evidence of therapeutic practices on the Highland mainland and the Western as well as the Northern Isles.

So far, the earliest known settlement site in Scotland is a Mesolithic one at Kinloch on the Isle of Rum[3] which dates to the mid-seventh millennium BC, but the pollen samples may reveal more about the then natural environment than the extent to which individual plants, shrubs and trees were used domestically and medicinally. Analytical techniques in archaeology have improved considerably over recent years, however, and it may not be long before the experts begin to learn much more about medicine in very ancient times.[4]

Given the natural 'pharmacy' that lay all around the homes and trails of our early ancestors, and the later known use of herbs, minerals, and creatures, it is only fair to attribute the subsequent wisdom and knowledge of medicine to the basis laid down in the Isle of Rum and elsewhere so many thousands of years ago.

The fact that Mesolithic settlers would have brought medical knowledge from their previous homelands, does not detract from their pioneering work in the country that was to become Scotland. In the Highlands, as the great glaciers retreated and scoured away traces of pre-Ice Age inhabitants, there would have been fauna and flora quite strange to the incomers. Patient experiments, doubtless a share of accidents both good and unfortunate, as well as occasional leaps of insight and genius, over the years would have evolved into a sound understanding of medicine, however primitive it may look by our standards.

The hunter/gatherer way of life of the earliest Highlanders may well have made up in quality of health what it appears to have lacked in longevity. It is also likely that abortion, infanticide and euthanasia as well as varyingly successful forms of contraception, known to be the custom of many peoples with a similar way of life, were practised by the Mesolithic people of the Highlands for the same reasons: the need for compact, healthy, easily controlled social groups. Population increases in itinerant tribes would have caused unwieldy logistical, hygienic and social problems. In hunter/gatherer times small groupings would have been the only viable social ones, even though food would have been no problem for such people living in the hills, glens and coastal plains of the north and the islands some 7000 years ago when the climate was more favourable than now and nature provided an abundance of nourishment.

They had salmon, shellfish, wild boar and venison, nuts, fruit and berries, root and leaf vegetables, as well as the purest of water supplies. At a reception given in the Royal Museum of Scotland in 1988 the food – salted hazelnuts, oatcakes with crowdie, watercress and herbs, brosemeal pancakes stuffed with mushrooms and juniper berries, smoked venison with a yoghurt and rowanberry dip, laverbread and oatmeal balls, smoked salmon in pumpernickel, and parsnip-and-carrot croquettes – was prepared only from raw materials available in the Highlands during the Mesolithic and early Neolithic periods, and very delicious it was, too. There is no telling that the prehistoric cooks would not have come up with equally well-presented and tasty morsels. After all, they would have had plenty of time to give to their art, and, thousands of years hence, who might tell simply from our well-rotted rubbish tips the complexities of our modern cuisine?

Because of the acidity of much of Scotland's soil, there is a lack of skeletal and other organic material from which to deduce a clearer picture of life in post-glacial settlement times. But since it is only in recent years that much attention at all has been paid to the Scottish Mesolithic period there may well be, somewhere, as yet undiscovered testimony to a fascinating chunk of Scotland's very distant past.

Consistently waterlogged sites help to preserve organic materials and the Highlands certainly abounds in bogs, lochs, pools and burns.

About 5500 years ago the customs of the earliest people began to give way to the agriculture and permanent settlements of the Neolithic period with its need for larger populations to tend the fields and livestock, harvest the crops and defend the inhabitants. They began to develop more structured social hierarchies, and the weapons that their forerunners had employed mainly for hunting became increasingly necessary to fend off human predators as more and more land became an object of possession.

Stone Age diets are often vaunted as a model for healthy eating with little account being taken of the wear and tear on teeth by coarsely-ground grains mixed with additives of powder and grit from the stone querns in which they were prepared. Teeth of this early agricultural period are often found to be heavily eroded, with a resulting 'box-like' arrangement – resembling that of children's milk-teeth – in adults. With the evenly ground spacing acting as a self-cleansing facility, caries were rare, but the inevitable exposure of the dental pulp in older adults meant that infections leading to abscesses were a constant danger, although surprisingly few abscesses appear to have caused any serious problems since they seem either to have cleared up spontaneously or with the help of some now lost treatment. In those unfortunates with jawbones badly decayed as the result of abscesses and, possibly, cancers, there is evidence that people could live for years or even decades with the consequences. And there is other evidence to show that their society was not the brutal, uncaring one of popular imagi-nation because people crippled in some way or other – and skeletal remains do not show the effects of many diseases and cancers that may have been present – are known to have lived for years with chronic disabilities. Such people, unable to hunt or labour in the fields, would have survived only with the help of their kin or caring neighbours.

Since Thomas Hobbes' remark on the life of man as 'solitary, poor, nasty, brutish and short' has been so persistently quoted out of context that it has by now become synonymous with the life of Stone Age people, it may be worth reminding readers that, although the words occur in the chapter of *Leviathan* headed 'Of the Natural Condition of Mankind', the phrase in question refers to man's lot in time of war and similar states of deep insecurity when it was, and sadly too often *is* today, impossible to cultivate the earth, construct great works – Carnac, Callanish, Stonehenge – and maintain social cohesion.

Some surgery was established by 2000 BC. An early Bronze Age trepanned skull found in the Island of Bute is evidence of a practice not only echoed in the procedures used by Neil Beaton of Husabost over 3500 years later, but in worldwide customs. Exactly why circular pieces of bone were carefully cut from the skull in prehistoric times continues to baffle experts. Was it for magical reasons – the releasing of evil spirits – or medical ones, or a combination of both? Martin noted of the Husabost empiric that 'he had the boldness to cut a piece out of a Woman's skull broader than half a Crown, and by this restored her to perfect Health'.

Trepanning or trephining for medical reasons was described by Hippocrates (460–377 BC) who is known to have scorned beliefs in 'evil spirits' as mere superstition. In the early twentieth century it was being practised in the South Pacific islands in cases of head-injuries caused by sling-stones. In almost every instance where it has been identified in ancient skulls the tricky operation had been skilfully carried out, often with a diagonal cut made into the bone presumably so that had the knife slipped it would have continued an upward curve, minimising the risk of injury to the brain. The operation is performed in modern surgery, mainly for the removal of splintered bone or foreign bodies such as bullets, and for the removal or relief of pressures caused by tumours.

Those who look with nostalgia on the natural medicines of our ancestors often leave surgery and dentistry out of the reckoning – though perhaps those puffball mushroom spores helped in some measure to alleviate the agonies.

Despite their Christian overlay, the toothache charms point to very early origins and the belief in sympathetic magic common to pre-industrial societies. Incantations collected orally in the nineteenth century have their parallels in those quoted in the Celtic writings of a thousand years before and are a glimpse into the understanding of spiritual dimensions of healing before, and parallel with, Christianity. One Gaelic incantation, a love charm rather than a healing one, involving the use of threads resembles one in a Latin poem written between 43 and 30 BC.

In C.H. Sisson's translation of Virgil's eighth Eclogue the jealous Alphesiboeus sings:

> My songs, bring Daphnis home again
> I pull three threads through you, three
> Of different colours, image, see
> For heaven is a trinity.
> My songs, bring Daphnis from the town
> And, Amaryllis, tie three knots
> And call them lovers' knots, for what
> Are three coloured knots if not that?[5]

Just over 1700 years later Thomas Pennant remarked, in his *A Tour in Scotland and Voyage to the Hebrides, 1772,* on a charm employed by a disappointed Highland lover:

> Donald takes three threads of different hues, and ties three knots of each, three times imprecating the most cruel disappointments on the nuptial bed . . .

Indeed, Virgil's whole Eclogue, with its references to sacred water, incantations, herbs, and the seducing of seeds 'silently from another's field', might be translated wholesale into Gaelic and mischievously passed off as purely Celtic.

In the 1970s and 1980s, I heard from acquaintances (see chapter 13) of *Eòlas an t-Snàithlein*, or the Charm of the Thread, still in use by healers in places as far apart as the Hebrides and Kiltarlity in Inverness-shire, although such practices were becoming increasingly rare. In 1982 I received a letter from Mary McGinley, a Scots nurse then working in the remote Chiriqui mountains of Panama, in which she described a ritual use of red threads as a protective charm for babies currently being employed by the Guayami Indians among whom she was living. It was astonishingly similar to those described by travellers in the Gaelic-speaking areas of Scotland from the late seventeenth century onwards.

It has been reasoned that such widespread traditions probably stem not so much from a basic culture that became dispersed throughout the world in mankind's very distant past as from patterns of instinctive human thinking common to us all but increasingly overlaid by what we call 'progress'. Sadly, the word 'primitive' has come to be popularly understood in the sense of something that is crude or ignorant rather than fundamental or simply 'original'. We mistakenly associate a lack of technological sophistication with a lack of intellect and insight. The ancients were as much aware of the forces of nature as we are, perhaps more so for they had fewer distractions, and just as we have built a complex language and system of mathematics around our understanding of the universe, so they constructed a mythology – except that they did not know it was a mythology. The gods, goddesses and emotions on which their universe turned was their knowledge, and a very human science that was essentially – in its origins, anyway – a humble one, recognising that humanity is so often at the mercy of stronger energies. Brigid[6], the Celtic goddess invoked in childbirth and many healing matters, and Dian Cécht, the god of medicine, must surely have originated as expressions of the human need for superhuman help and the drive to define and understand the stranger forces of creation.

Comparisons may be made between the legends of the Gaels and those of the ancient Greeks and other societies which show how closely the early, less culturally cluttered human intellect identified healing with the sacred and a sense of destiny. The adventures of Hercules and Jason, whose name means 'healer', are reflected in such early Gaelic tales as 'The Fate of the Children of Tuirenn' who are sent on quests whose objects include three apples from the Gardens of the Hesperides which when eaten remedy diseases and wounds and promptly return to their whole state to await another cure; a pigskin renowned for healing all ills; and the hound-whelp of the king of Ioruaidhe which echoes the dog associated with the Greek god of healing, Asclepius.

The goddess Brigid and her Christian 'successor' St Brigid of Kildare have so many aspects and legends in common that the two are virtually inextricable. Thus it was doubtless meant to be, and the question will be explored in Chapter 3. Of more immediate interest is the fact that Brigid represents one of the furthest reaching threads of all.

The Romans, who had the happy knack of assimilating 'barbarian' deities to the nearest equivalent in their own pantheon, saw in Brigantia, the mainland British counterpart of Brigid, the attributes of their own Minerva. In their turn the Romans had adopted Minerva from the wise Athene of the Greeks, who owed much to the Egyptian concept of Isis. Behind all these seems to lie the influence of the Libyan snake-goddess, Neit. Like Brigid and her classical parallels, Neit was a protectress of women and childbirth, marriage, the arts and domestic skills. Taken up by the Egyptians as the guardian of their city of Saïs, a school of medicine, called the House of Life, was annexed to her sanctuary. In the Libyan cosmogony she was the Celestial Cow who gave birth to the sky, and as the supreme weaver she wove the world with her shuttle. Brigid, too, was closely associated with spinning, weaving and cattle as well as healing.

Whether into all this warp and weft can be read a strong early dissemination of medical knowledge and philosophy, it would be dangerous to say, but this much is certain: just as in the Middle Ages when the Gaelic practice of medicine was to be firmly rooted in the mainstream of western European orthodox medicine while at the same time paying due respect to its native heritage, so from the very earliest times it appears to have absorbed, and probably helped to generate, a steady stream of intercultural ideas. In a paper read to the Gaelic Society of Inverness in 1924, the Revd Angus MacFarlane remarked: 'It may be questioned if there are any of the great races of mankind so widely versed in the curative values of plants and herbs as the Celts, except the American Indian.' To which he might have added the Chinese who have the benefit of written records going back thousands of years, but the point is well made. The Celts, both continental and insular, in their turn owed much to their aboriginal predecessors. The mushrooms of Skara Brae were, so to speak, to spread their spores far and wide.

2

MAGICAL WATER AND SMELLY ONIONS

Down the ages the purity of the water supply was a vital asset in maintaining health in the Highlands and it has even been suggested that the abundance of holy wells and springs dedicated to various saints stemmed from an early recognition of the importance of clean water. However, it is doubtful whether a lack of unpolluted sources – though problems may have been caused by the widespread effect of the enormous eruption of Mount Hekla in Iceland in about 1150 BC – in the Bronze Age alone led to people's penchant in that period for depositing valuable votive offerings in pools or rivers. The practice swept Scotland from the end of the third millennium to about 500 BC, and it hints strongly at a respect for the guardian spirits, gods, or whatever the concept was, of the waters.[1]

The likeliest interpretation is that purity of water was a recognised necessity for good health, but that alongside this certain waters were found to contain a specific remedial property, and yet others were simply appealing because of their situation in the landscape or because of association with happy events. Sulphur or chalybeate springs did not, after all, suddenly appear from nowhere to suit the whims of the early nineteenth century. When we think about ancient medicine we tend to give it a herbal association, but the fact is that just about everything from the light-reflecting crystal and the magnificent antler of the stag to the everyday banality of dung and cobwebs was experimented with for its curative powers. It would have been more amazing if water had been left out of the reckoning. Equally, a sense of 'spirit of place' and an appreciation of even the smallest details of nature were a distinct feature of early Gaelic and other Celtic cultures long before the eighteenth century Romantic movement brought the delights of the countryside to the attention of a largely urbanised European art and literature.[2]

Long before the coming of scientific methods of testing water, people learned from experience, both good and bad, of the qualities of streams and wells. Explanations of how some springs came to lose their power by people using them for washing dirty hands or taking dogs or other beasts to drink at them may reflect ancient taboos against offending the spirits of the waters – in our terms: causing pollution.

Of Bronze Age medicine in the Highlands little is known save for that trephined skull found in Bute, but it is fair to suppose that a period which saw great advances in metallurgy, both practical and ornamental, the proliferation of extraordinary stone monuments and a growth in trade with Continental Europe as far, at least, as the Mediterranean, would also have seen advances in medicine. A society which gave tens of thousands of man hours to raising, for example, the Ring of Brodgar in Orkney, or Callanish in Lewis[3], would hardly have resented comparable time being spent on research into curing disease.

For all the lack of material evidence for medical practices, the Bronze Age was a seminal period for Highland traditions. The water, the metal, the stones, and the magical powers associated with the people who worked them – the miller and the boatman, the black-smith, the mason – were to remain enduring features of the culture for thousands of years. Organic materials such as herbs are harder to pin down, but it seems feasible that the women who were responsible for so much in field and home were also shrewd investigators of the remedial properties of the natural world.

Women had a high status in ancient medicine, as Mediterranean mythology bears witness. North-west Europe is far less well endowed with written evidence for the times, but a Bronze Age site in Denmark, described by P.V. Glob in *The Mound People*, tells an interesting story:

> A site at Maglehoj in the west part of north Zealand, excavated by Vilhelm Boye in 1888, shows that women also took over the role of medicine man. At the bottom of the mound stood a small stone coffin covered with a heavy block of stone, eel-grass and a heap of stones that had protected the grave from earth sifting down. Inside was a woman's belt box, a double-headed fastener, a knife and a fibula of bronze on top of the cremated bones, which had been wrapped in a piece of woollen clothing. Within the bronze box – of a kind that women carried on their backs – were the sorcerer's charms: two horse's teeth, some weasel (marten) bones, the claw-joint of a member of the cat family (possibly a lynx), bones from a young mammal (a lamb or a deer), a piece less than half an inch long of a bird's windpipe, some vertebrae from a snake, two burnt fragments of bone (human?), a twig of mountain ash, charred aspen, two pebbles of quartz, a lump of clay, two pieces of pyrites, a sheet of bronze, and a piece of bronze wire bent at one end to form a small hook. Both the belt-fastener and the bronze box were ornamented with star patterns.[4]

This medicine-woman's box of tricks may be compared with the *pocan cheann*, bag of heads, still kept in the Highlands into the present century, which contained the heads of an adder, a toad and a newt and was used for healing. The *pocan* was dipped in a stream which divided two crofts and the water which escaped from the bag when lifted was applied to the wound. Yet another comparison might be made with the curious tools of trade kept by the eighteenth-century woman known as Fitheach, the 'witch' of Ballachly near Rangag in the Caithness parish of Latheron. She lived in a turf hut close to the cemetery and no one knew where she came from, or even what her true name was. In this bothy she kept an assortment of strange objects, so placed as to be in the full view of, and presumably impress with her powers, anyone that might happen to visit her. There were unusually shaped stones, rough clay urns, wooden cups, hair ropes, dried cabbage runts, bladders full of ravens' feathers, and cow's hair kept in a small case or straw basket.[5]

Glob also remarked:

> . . . in the late Bronze Age, female deities assumed a prominent place among the male gods until they actually came to dominate. This may be clearly seen in late Bronze Age representations from Denmark and is reflected in the sacrificial objects placed beside sacred springs and elsewhere in earth and fen. For whereas the objects sacrificed at the beginning of the Bronze Age consisted exclusively of weapons and other gifts to male divinities, women's ornaments and associated items gradually replaced them almost entirely in the sacrificial groves of the late Bronze Age.[6]

It is a far cry from the female deities of the Bronze Age to the witch of Ballachly's lowly hut and her uncomplimentary sobriquet of Fitheach, which means 'raven', a bird of ill omen. In her *Old Wives' Tales: Their History, Remedies and Spells*, Mary Chamberlain makes a telling and pithy comment: 'Old wives began as goddesses but ended as back-street abortionists'.[7]

Tacitus makes some interesting remarks about the Iron Age tribes of Germany which may have been applicable further afield in the north-west:

> It is to their mothers and wives that they go to have their wounds treated, and the women are not afraid to count and compare the gashes.[8]

Then there is Tacitus' report of the German womenfolk on the battlefield:

> It stands on record that armies already wavering and on the point of collapse have been rallied by the women, pleading heroically with their men, thrusting forward their bared bosoms, and making them realise the imminent prospect of enslavement.

This compares with his remarks (below) on what may have been a branch of female druids in Anglesey. The idea of women working on an intellectual, as opposed to domestic, level alongside druids is often neglected, perhaps because our notion of the latter is still fixed by the writings and prejudices of male antiquarians from the seventeenth century onwards. Until quite recently 'doctor' or 'lawyer' implied a man, so why not a druid, too, seems to have been the assumption. Yet in *The Annals of Imperial Rome* Tacitus clearly describes a vociferous caste of black-clad women who may have been the female counterpart of the male priesthood if not an independent grouping of similar potency.

A Roman force under Suetonius Paulinus was sent to attack the druidic sanctuary of Mona (Anglesey) in AD 60, and arrived on the island to an awesome demonstration from its inhabitants which cowed even that campaigned-hardened and disciplined army:

> The enemy lined the shore in a dense armed mass. Among them were black-robed women with dishevelled hair like Furies, brandishing torches. Close by stood Druids, raising their hands to heaven and screaming dreadful curses. The weird spectacle awed the Roman soldiers into a sort of paralysis. They stood still – and presented themselves as a target. But then they urged each other (and were urged by the general) not to fear a horde of fanatical women. Onward pressed their standards and they bore down their opponents, enveloping them in the flames of their own torches. Suetonius garrisoned the conquered island. The groves devoted to Mona's barbarous superstitions he demolished.[9]

In her *Pagan Celtic Britain*, Anne Ross sees the Mona women as 'an echo of the black-raven goddesses, depriving their enemies of their strength and valour through their magic posture and incantation, and rushing among the troops prophesying the outcome of the fight and the doom of the heroes'.[10] In his rigorous exploration of druidic fact and fiction, *The Druids*, Stuart Piggott writes of the name 'druid' lingering on after the Roman abolition of the sect, in the 'debased sense of a magician or prophet . . . as the stories about the prophecies made by *female Druids* to Alexander Severus, Diocletian and Aurelian show'.[11] (My italics.) Irish mythology tells of several raven or crow-goddesses closely associated both with battles and water. The name given to that poor old woman of Ballachly may well have been a lingering vestige of a very old folk-memory, and it is interesting that she appears even to have encouraged her weird reputation.

It is even possible to connect a Gaelic goddess, a battle and knowledge of healing herbs. The story also shows that professional jealousy of women and other healers by the medical establishment probably had a very long history.

In the First Battle of Moytura, so the story goes, the hand of Nuada, leader of the Tuatha Dé Danann[12], was cut off in battle. The smith Credne Cerd made a silver one so skilfully that all its joints moved. After it was fitted by Dian Cécht, the Gaelic Asclepius, the leader was known as Nuada *Argetlám*, 'Silverhand'. For all its strength, beauty and agility, however, the false hand was a false hand and since, according to Celtic custom, no maimed person might rule, Nuada was removed from power. During the crisis provoked by the need to find a new leader, who should turn up on Nuada's doorstep but Miach and Airmedh, the son and daughter of Dian Cécht. After impressing the half-blind doorkeeper by replacing his bad eye with a good one from a cat[13], they easily gained access to Nuada himself, whom they found tormented by an infection where the silver hand joined the flesh.

Miach had Nuada's own long-since buried hand dug up and placed it on the stump. Over it Miach chanted one of the best-known of the old Gaelic charms, enjoining each sinew, each nerve, each vein and each bone to reunite, and in three days the hand and arm were as if they had never been parted, with feeling and deftness of touch in every finger. (The Celts were never averse to exaggeration.)

Dian Cécht was furious that his son should thus be shown to be the superior physician, and after various attacks which Miach survived through healing himself, his father finally cleft his brain in two during the Second Battle of Moytura. But even the dead Miach was not quite finished. Out of his grave there grew 365 herbs, each a specific for healing the part of the body from which it sprang. Airmedh picked each herb and laid it on her outspread cloak according to the part of the body where it had grown so that she might remember its healing property. Unfortunately, Dian Cécht, angry and jealous as ever, could not cope with the idea of his daughter gaining such knowledge, and in a fit of temper shook up the mantle and completely muddled its contents. Were it not for such pettiness, we should have known how to cure every ill, including death itself, or so the story went.

But what of the thwarted Airmedh? The old chroniclers were not so interested in her story and turned again to the politics and the battles. It might be reasoned that, since she was clever enough to sort the herbs systematically and fortunate enough to have accompanied her gifted brother on his healing missions, she was well-enough equipped to carry on her researches and practice of medicine. Doubtless, this mythical forerunner of the henwife would have had a vivid memory of those herbs on the cloak and the ability to fill in the gaps by experiment. What this shrewd lady of her times most certainly would have done was to have been discreet about her knowledge with her competitive father hovering in the background, and doubtless a body of male druids also on the look-out for uppity females.

It is not, perhaps, unreasonable to read into this legend a parallel female healing tradition which dealt essentially in practical matters handed down orally from generation to generation, while male healers developed theories and ethics along professional lines. To this day mothers and wives retain a considerable knowledge of first-aid methods that seems to materialise when needed almost by a process of osmosis.

In comparison with much of Europe at the time, the Iron Age Celts and Picts of the north seem to have had a relatively stable existence. For one thing there is far more evidence of inward rather than outward migration, suggesting a place worth fleeing to for peace and general survival – if the natives were willing. The Romans were repulsed to the southern side of Antonine's Wall, the Anglians were vanquished at the battle of Dunnichen (or Nechtansmere as it was known to invaders). It was not until later incursions, first by Irish Gaels and later by the Vikings that major cultural alterations occurred.

The Iron Age peoples of the north were above all farmers. The Picts[14], in particular, settled in the better agricultural areas and are known to have been sound builders and traders. Their economy was stable enough to allow a magnificent outpouring of art, remains of which can still be seen in the shape of their superb stone-carvings and jewellery and the inspiration they provided for designs in Christian works such as the Book of Kells.

From what is known of skeletal material, the Picts seem to have been a fit people, although there is some evidence of arthritis and leprosy and, like earlier peoples, their teeth were well worn by a diet of rough grains and tough meat. As likely as not, their daily life and diet was much like that of the people who were less debatably recorded as Celts and Gaels. But call the Iron Age inhabitants of the north what we will, they lived in a society which relished its feasting and drinking, especially the latter. The Celtic knowledge of brewing intrigued the Romans and in one small herb, the tuberous vetch, there is a link between notes on its use by the Celts in the writings of Dioscorides, Athenaeus (quoting Posidonius), Julius Caesar and Cassius Dio, and its similar use in the Highlands up to nearly 2000 years later for the same reasons – allaying hunger and flavouring alcoholic drinks.

Although the tasty tubers of the plant were once roasted and eaten like chestnuts in Holland and Flanders, its use as noted by the Romans appears to have been uniquely Celtic. Current quibbles among archaeologists as to whether the continental and insular Celts can be said to have had similar material cultures, or whether the early insular Iron Age peoples can be said to be Celts at all, might take a different turn if herbal traditions were taken into account alongside other factors.

Plant remedies attributed by Pliny, for one, to the Gauls and their druids appear in the medicinal lore of the Gaels and the Welsh, as well as in other Western European folk traditions. The uses and historical records of the tuberous vetch are discussed in Chapter 14.

The Iron Age diet seems to have been a good and varied one. Protein came from dairy produce, an abundance of fish such as salmon and trout, wildfowl and the meat of deer, cattle, goats, sheep and boar. A wide range of vegetables and herbs was eaten, both cooked and in salads. Watercress was popular as were parsnips and seaweeds, carrots and leafy vegetables. Culinary skills were sophisticated. Anne Ross explains in her *Everyday Life of the Pagan Celts* how, according to early Irish texts, salmon was baked with honey and herbs, and Athenaeus refers to other fish cooked with salt, vinegar and cumin.[15] And there was corn, especially barley, aplenty, although the cultivated oats that were to become the mainstay of the later Scottish diet were first introduced to southern Britain by the Romans.

Since it is largely a good balanced diet that enables people to fulfil their growth potential it is no surprise to find – from skeletal remains – that, far from being the stunted 'fairy'-like folk of legends, the Picts were not far from the average height of present-day Scots. In 563 St Columba, or Calum Cille as he is known in Scottish Gaelic, arrived in Scotland with his mission to convert the northern Picts as St Ninian had worked with the southern Picts about a century earlier. Since the story of Calum Cille belongs properly to that of the influence of the church on medicine it will be dealt with in the next chapter. The 'threads' should be elastic enough here to leap to the time of the Vikings in Scotland – from the end of the eighth century.

The particular influence of the Norse on Gaelic medicine, and vice versa, is hard to gauge, they share similar healing legends, the same peripheral position in Europe and much of the same natural medicinal sources. However, strong Scandinavian links with the Arab world via the trade routes to Constantinople and beyond, suggest that these, as much as direct links between the Arab world and southern Ireland, introduced what was to re-emerge as a fondness for the Arabian approach to medicine, with its emphasis on research and experiment.

Ibn Fadlan, ambassador of the Caliph of Baghdad, travelled extensively among the Rus people of Scandinavia in the early tenth century and wrote graphically of what he saw. His narrative was followed some years later by the writings of Ibn Rustah. The constant interaction between Arab and Scandinavian, Scandinavian and Hiberno-Scottish Gael and both these latter with the Picts made not only for territorial and political skirmishes but also for a rich cultural broth.

As with Tacitus' story of the German women treating the wounded on the battlefield, Snorri's *Saga of King Harald* tells how women heated, possibly even sterilised, water to clean wounds which they then dressed. What well may have been the first diagnostic meal, in the latter half of the ninth century, was prepared from a mess of onions and herbs and fed to those with severe abdominal wounds. After a while, the medical attendant would lean over and sniff at the man's belly. If the reek of onions could be detected around the injury, it meant only one thing – the intestines had been damaged and the man would be given up for dead. The fatally wounded would then be left, perhaps with some painkilling draught, while those more likely to recover would receive what attention could be given. It was a hard world.

A proper sense of hygiene is often believed to have been introduced to these islands, via southern Britain, by the Romans and to have disappeared for many centuries after the Roman withdrawal. However, the likely use of what archaeologists call 'burnt mound sites' as washing, sauna and hydrotherapy as well as cooking areas (see Chapter 10) and the discovery of drainage systems in domestic sites, such as the Ardestie souterrain in Angus, tell a rather different tale. Medicated baths are often mentioned in early Gaelic literature. In the *Táin Bó Cúailnge* (Great Cattle Raid of Cooley) Conchobhar's physician Fingen uses a bath of herbs medicated with the marrow of cows. Other sources tell of baths in the milk of 150 white hornless cattle or in water infused with the qualities of various herbs. There are also mentions of taking baths for the cure of leprosy and other skin diseases.

The Vikings, who were also far cleaner than their popular image allows, would have introduced their regular Saturday custom, the *laugardagr*, or bath day. According to an early literary source quoted by Johannes Brønsted in *The Vikings*, the Danes also combed their hair and changed their linen frequently 'in order the more easily to overcome the chastity of women and procure the daughters of noblemen as their mistresses'.[16] If their close-fitting helmets and bristling fur jerkins procured rather more irritating close relationships, with fleas and lice, then they had regular, almost ritual, de-lousing sessions.

3

MONKS AND MEDICINE

The influence of the Christian church on Gaelic medicine in Scotland may be matched by the influence of the native tradition on the Celtic church itself. Again, the threads interweave. From the arrival of Calum Cille[1] in 563 to the burning of Iona by the Vikings in 802, the Highlands saw a great flowering of art and culture. Even the acceptance by the greater part of the Celtic church of the authority of Rome at the Synod of Whitby in 664, which triggered the erosion of insular Celtic autonomy (or symptomised the end of insular Celtic isolation), would have had little effect on the workings of the specifically healing side of the mission.

The native religion that Calum Cille found among the Picts remains a matter for speculation but was probably similar to that of other north-west Celtic Iron Age beliefs with a strong base in the natural world and the observable universe and its interaction with humanity. Although the mission of converting the Picts to Christianity was not fully accomplished in Calum Cille's own lifetime, the fact that progress was relatively uncomplicated if not entirely without its setbacks, may owe something to a recognition by the Picts that the new religion was an *improvement* on their current beliefs rather than a totally strange set of concepts. This may also have been why the early Celtic church found it easy to assimilate elements of the old pagan ways into their own practice. Much the same picture might be applied to the physical remedies the missionaries introduced.

Adomnán, the biographer of Calum Cille, records that when the saint visited the northern pagan Pictish king Bridei (or Brude) at his court near Inverness, the king, after initial haughtiness, 'throughout the rest of his life, greatly honoured the holy and venerable man, as was fitting, with high esteem'.[2] Bridei's high druid, Broichan, however, was a tougher proposition and professional jealousy and pride – both religious and medical – may have been involved.

Calum Cille begged Broichan to free a young woman slave but the druid stubbornly refused to part with her, whereupon the saint told Broichan, in the presence of the king, that he (the druid) would die before Calum Cille himself left the area. The saint then left the court and went to the river Ness from which he took a white pebble. On showing it to his companions he said:

> Mark this white stone. Through it the Lord will work many cures of the sick among this heathen people . . . Now Broichan has received a hard blow. For an angel sent from heaven has struck him heavily, and broken into many pieces in his hand the glass vessel from which he was drinking, and has left him breathing with difficulty, and near to death. Let us wait a little in this place for two messengers of the king, sent to us in haste, to obtain our immediate help for the dying Broichan. Now Broichan, terribly stricken, is ready to release the slave-girl.[3]

Before Calum Cille had finished speaking two horsemen arrived to relate how everything had occurred according to the prediction. The blessed pebble was then taken to the king by two of the saint's companions who had been assured: 'If first Broichan promises that he will release the slave-girl, then let this small stone be dipped in water, and let him drink thereof and he will at once recover health. But if he refuses, and opposes the slave-girl's release, he will immediately die.'

Whatever Adomnán's penchant for stretching credibility in his wish to put across his hero as a miracle-worker, seer, and general spiritual prodigy, it is possible to see here Calum Cille's strength and shrewdness in playing on the druids' superstitions and psychic snobbery. In Calum Cille, Broichan had met more than his match. Needless to say, the king and his druid released the slave to the saint's messengers, and when Broichan drank from the water on which the pebble mysteriously floated, he was instantly healed.

The story goes on to tell how the pebble was kept among the king's treasures and was often used for curing a range of diseases. If a person's 'time had come', however, the stone could not be found, and on the day Bridei died the pebble was missing from the place where it was carefully kept. Such a stress on the healing power of stones was to be retained for many centuries in the Highlands, and where elsewhere rock crystal balls, for instance, were endowed with the power of foretelling the future, they rarely had this supposed attribute among the Gaels. As will be seen in Chapter 11, the rock crystal was, above all, assumed to be a medium of healing. Broichan turned out to be remarkably ungrateful for his miracle cure and carried out a threat to raise a violent storm on Loch Ness as Calum Cille and his party set sail for the south. The holy man, according to Adomnán, countered this by turning the wind into a favourable light breeze. Broichan had called upon his pagan deities, Calum Cille his Christian one. The common folk of the Picts were to be left in no doubt as to where the stronger power lay.

Not surprisingly, virtually all Calum Cille's cures recorded by Adomnán are in the field of spiritual or psychological healing and need not necessarily be regarded as a figment of Adomnán's proselytising quill. Faith can be a powerful healer and, even allowing for his biographer's zeal, Calum Cille comes across as a man of extraordinary influence. Moreover, 80–90 per cent of physical illnesses clear up on their own account. A shrewd sense of the workings of the human mind on the human body was ever a part of the Gaelic medical tradition. When the human mind was elevated by a strong belief in the divine, and when that Christian divinity was synonymous with the most powerful of human emotions, love, the potential for healing was heady indeed.

The Columban mission aimed to convert the old druidic system of divination and astrology into a Christianised version of divinely inspired revelation and a fate in the hands of a loving God rather than a wilful universe. Pagan Celtic incantations became rather more thinly disguised as prayers. The old deities of the waters gave way to saintly protectors. It worked up to a point and certainly a potent belief in the old goddess Brigid appears to have had a relatively smooth metamorphosis into St Brigid.

The Christian Brigid (c. 452–524) was the daughter of an Ulster slavewoman and was in turn sold as a slave to a druid whom she won over to Christianity by her own gentle goodness. Twenty years after becoming a nun she founded a mixed community of monks and nuns at Kildare, south of Dublin, not far from the ancient site of Dun Ailinn which may have been a centre for the cult of her pagan namesake. It is interesting that a perpetual flame tended by nineteen nuns, until it was extinguished during the Reformation, is a distinct echo of the perpetual fire tended by nineteen virgins at the goddess's shrine. In the twelfth century, Geraldus of Wales wrote that no male was allowed to enter the sacred enclosure where the fire burned, again, perhaps, a reversion to a pagan priestess cult. Both goddess and saint were ascribed the same attributes as protectors of women in childbirth and scholars at their studies, and both were patrons of the arts and poetry and domestic skills.

There is no record of St Brigid having visited Scotland but early church and place-name dedications are numerous here. There are Kilbrides in, among other areas, Lanarkshire, Ayrshire, Argyll, South Uist and Skye and a number of healing wells are dedicated to her. An indigenous mother goddess, like her Irish counterpart, was apparently easily assimilated into the figure of St Brigid.

For all the accent on the heightened mystical side of the healing mission, purely practical matters were not ignored. Calum Cille is recorded as having been consulted about nosebleeds and fractures and he was especially resorted to for cures for blindness. There is some likelihood that the saint's reputation for ophthalmic 'miracles' may have been due to the monks' competence in using surgical couching for cataracts. The monks are known to have performed surgery. When a trephining of the skull was carried out in Ireland in 637 by St Bricin, the scribe noted that the 'brain of forgetfulness was removed' from the patient, Cennfaeladh, that is, the portion of the skull that had been injured in battle and was deemed to be causing lethargy.

The missionaries also had some clever ways with herbs. One practice which may have been new to the northern Picts has been passed down through the centuries in the Gaelic name of a common moorland plant, the St John's wort or *achlasan Chaluim Chille*. The Gaelic term is rather curious and literally translates into English as St Columba's oxterful. A traditional story is told of how a young herd boy whose nerves had been upset by long dark, lonely nights out in the hills with the cattle, was brought to the saint for a cure for his condition. Calum Cille is said to have placed the St John's wort in the boy's armpit, whereupon he began to recover his balance of mind. The story and the name of the plant are so specific that they must surely relate to poultices placed by monastic healers in patients' armpits, that part of the body – like the groin – being so well endowed with nerve-endings, glands and blood vessels that it readily absorbs substances into the body's system as a whole. There were no hypodermic needles in those days, so a form of inunction, absorption of medicament through the skin, would have been practised. It is now known that St John's wort contains rutin which affects the flow of adrenalin which in turn influences the sympathetic nervous system. A later folk cure for pneumonia which involved placing an onion in each oxter would also have stemmed from the belief in inunction.

In *Sages, Saints and Storytellers: Celtic Studies in honour of Professor James Carney*, Wendy Davies' contribution on 'The Place of Healing in Early Irish Society' contains a table which compares the proportion of specifically *healing* miracles in nine Lives of Celtic saints. It is clear from this that for the five male saints only up to nine per cent of their miracles were of a healing nature, but in the case of the four female Lives the proportion rises to seventeen per cent in the case of St Ita and forty per cent for St Brigid, a likely indication that healing was very much a female province. Davies suggests that this was because of the low status of healing; yet, surely, as Ronald Black has pointed out in a review of the book, it speaks more of the 'relatively high status of women' in that society. As the influence of the wider Christian church and European culture as a whole encroached on that of the Celts, the role of women in medicine became an increasingly peripheral and alternative one. Some indication of the importance of lay and female healers, however, may be derived from scanning the records of medieval hospices in the Highland area.

The major practical achievement of the church regarding medicine in Scotland was the founding of hospitals.[4] Early establishments would have been very small in comparison with later ones and they were inevitably attached to monastic settlements. Evidence for such hospices in the Highlands is rare and only on the fringes of the area, and tends to date from the twelfth century onwards, although Ospisdale in east Sutherland with its Norse suffix may suggest a Celtic foundation resettled in Viking times. Could it be that, aside from a generally good standard of health and minimal contact with urban epidemics, the practice of Gaelic community and domestic care was more than adequate for its time? The Gaels of later centuries who, by necessity, were forced to rely on traditional medicine, seem to have managed very well until wider contacts introduced disease (including new strains) on a scale which was beyond the scope of old methods.

In the Middle Ages the dominance of the church in healing inevitably led to theories not so much of medical ethics but of medicine's place in Christian doctrine. If God was all-loving then sickness and disease must be the result of sin, not forgetting the 'sins of the fathers' being visited on subsequent generations of children. Theologians pondered not only the number of dancing angels who might be accommodated on the point of a needle, but also whether or not the bowels moved in paradise or whether Adam and Eve had navels. So conservative were these men that they even frowned on the use of spectacles and forks on the grounds that the good Lord had provided both eyes and fingers.

However, the Celtic monks who had fled to the Continent in the wake, or in advance, of Norse raids, could never quite divorce themselves from their roots. The margins of several Latin manuscripts are peppered with references to pre-Christian cures and incantations, some of which refer to the Gaelic pagan god of medicine, Dian Cécht. (Examples are given in Chapter 13.)

In their Continental mission, these Celtic monks would have spread the practical as well as the spiritual element of their healing, and while we have no detailed record of the herb garden kept at Iona prior to the first Viking raids of the late eighth century, some idea of its range may be obtained from a record of the herb garden at St Gall in Switzerland, founded by the followers of the Irish monk Columbanus in 720. In a plan of the monastery and hospital garden made about a hundred years later, over thirty herbs and vegetables are listed: lilies, roses, climbing beans, pepperwort, costmary, fenugreek, rosemary, mint, sage, rue, iris, pennyroyal, watercress, cumin, lovage, fennel, onion-leaf celery, coriander, dill, poppies (including the opium variety), radishes, beet, garlic, shallots, parsley, chervil, lettuce, parsnip and cabbage. The dedicated work of the archaeo-botanist Brian Moffat at the medieval Augustinian hospice site at Soutra in the Lammermuir Hills, has revealed remains of very similar plants being used in a Lowland context.

After the Reformation a number of practices with Catholic connotations became absorbed into the general healing folklore of the Gaels alongside the older pagan ones. Charms were considered particularly efficacious if written on the consecrated vellum of a religious book. In unofficial medicine these charms were known as a *soisgeul* (gospel) and one tale is told of Fr Archibald Chisholm, a young priest in Glencoe, who was perplexed by some dozen Protestants applying to him in January 1840 for gospels to cure various illnesses.

This may be compared with the use of quite obviously pagan rituals and charms by people in the more staunchly presbyterian areas of the Western Isles in quite recent times. Despite a vigorous disapproval of 'superstition' by generations of Free Church ministers, many of their parishioners may see no inconsistency. Time and again my queries have received much the same amused response: 'But it's nothing to do with religion.' People would no more think of an association between a charm for the healing of broken bones and a Free Church metrical psalm, than they would of a link between a National Health Service prescription and a quotation from the Book of Leviticus.

Wells may have become associated with the names of saints but the days on which the wells were most resorted to were not the saints' feast-days but the old pagan quarter-days. Rituals for epilepsy, such as the one described in Chapter 6, might involve no end of strange procedures including drinking from a suicide's skull and being rowed sunwise around a loch, but none of this was seen by the people as incompatible with their deeply held Christianity.

This ability to harmonise what elsewhere became matters of conflict, culminating in the witchcraft trials of later centuries, may owe not a little to the understanding of the old ways by those Celtic missionaries, and the respect for that early Church engendered in the memory of countless generations of lay people.

The Gaels probably also introduced the Picts to the ancient Irish legal system, the Brehon Laws, which contained a tract on sick-maintenance including medicines, midwifery, epilepsy, removal of a joint or sinew, blood-letting, diet and tuberculosis. The Brehon ruling on hospitals alone shows a highly developed and caring society. They were, among other things, to have well-qualified doctors and attendants, to be free from debt, to have a plentiful supply of fresh water and to have their doors ever open for the free treatment of the sick be they old, widows, orphans, or in any way disadvantaged or distressed. As a whole, the Brehon Laws were a grand example of a well-structured society attempting to define the last jot and tittle of possible human behaviour and misbehaviour. Boasting of sexual prowess to someone other than a marriage partner, for instance, could give a woman, or a man, one of many grounds for divorce, though a husband might freely kiss and hug another man's wife on festive occasions (doing likewise on an ordinary day would cost him a fine). The early church protested at the divorce laws but made little headway in disturbing a system claimed to have been founded in 714 BC. In parts of Ireland the Laws were to survive until they were finally suppressed by the English in the mid-seventeenth century.

The care of the sick and the poor in the Gaelic tradition then, having been legislated for long before anyone thought of a Welfare State, was the responsibility of the community and the kindred or clan. In the Scottish Highlands and western islands this admirable tradition was to pave the way for a unique clan medical structure in the later Middle Ages. It is said to have begun with yet another Irish influx of learning, which this time accompanied not a political, military or religious mission – but a wedding party.

4

CLAN PATRONAGE AND
MEDIEVAL MEDICINE

Towards the end of the thirteenth century Áine (Agnes), a daughter of Cú-maige nan Gall Ó Catháin of Connacht, married Angus Og, Lord of the Isles. Tradition maintains that she brought from Ireland as her tocher, or dowry, a great retinue of men which consisted of 'seven score men out of every surname under O'Kain' from which sprang twenty-four families in Scotland. Among these families was listed a contingent of the medical kindred Mac Meic-bethad, later to be known as the MacBeths or, from the sixteenth century, Beatons.[1] This kindred was to flourish in Highland medicine for some 400 years, with at least nineteen branches of the family practising throughout the islands and the mainland as far south and east as Angus.[2] Yet to see them and the other Gaelic medical kindreds as bursting upon the Highland healing scene like astronauts among aliens would be far from realistic. Rather, the Irish tocher might be seen as an infusion of new blood and ideas which blended with the old, enabling Highland medicine to develop Irish as well as native theories and practices alongside the orthodox European system in the dynamic climate of the Renaissance.

The citing of genealogies and attendant legends in order to establish one's bona fides within a given social order was a favourite Gaelic pastime, and the Macbeths seem to have been adept at arranging their genealogy to fit the climate of any given time or place. It also suited them, when the need arose, to lay claim to roots in Fife and France, and legends and other details associate them, in folk memory at least, with the Norse and the Picts. Their European education may have led to opportunities for marrying Continental wives thus broadening the family connections of the physicians.

Interaction and communication between the Irish and the people of Alba, as Scotland is still called in Gaelic, are now known to have prevailed long before the colonisation of Argyll by the Irish *Scotti* was accomplished in the fifth century AD. Diseases and their cures tend to spread along the same routes, and next to germs few things travel faster than news or hope of a cure. The story told by the influential sixteenth-century Scots historian (and Gaelic-speaker) George Buchanan of a second century BC 'ninth King of Scotland' that he was educated in Ireland by native physicians and wrote a treatise on the use of herbs, may be somewhat ingenious, but it is true enough in spirit to the interests of later Scots rulers and nobility who considered medicine and science very proper studies and pastimes.

Among entries of assignments of land written into the ninth century Book of Deer in the early twelfth century, are those which appear to hint at a Pictish branch of the Mac Meic-bethad. The land for the monastery of Deer is said to have been donated to Calum Cille by '*Bede, Cruthnec ro bo mor maer Buchan*' (Bede, a Pict, who was high steward of Buchan). Elsewhere in the manuscript a Maldomni mac Meic Bead is mentioned as witness to a grant of lands to the monastery; and Donchad mac mec Bead Mec Hidid gave the lands of Achmachar 'free of all imposts for all time to Christ and to Drostan and to Colum Cille'. In his paper 'The MacBeths – Hereditary Physicians of the Highlands'[3] Alexander Nicolson points out: 'In commenting on the efforts made by King Alexander I of Scotland to restore order among his subjects, the writer of the Wardlaw MS states that " . . . the king created 'Donald Beaton' as governor of the castle of Dingwall in 1110."' At the same time such connections are extremely vague, and there were at least two others called Mac Meic-bethad in Ireland who had no obvious connection with hereditary medical practice. No evidence of a link between the forename of MacBeth, King of Scots, and the medical kindreds has ever been found, let alone claimed in even the most imaginative of the genealogies.

Such names may be coincidences or may even point to a 'trade' as well as a family name. The medieval Gaelic medical manuscripts cite Hippocrates more than any other source and it is worth noting that part of his famous Oath reads:

> I will pay the same respect to my master in the Science as to my parents and share my life with him and pay all my debts to him. I will regard his sons as my brothers and teach them the Science, if they desire to learn it, without fee or contract. I will hand on precepts, lectures and all other learning to my sons, to those of my master and to those pupils duly apprenticed and sworn, and to none other.

The Beatons as well as other Gaelic medical kindreds may well have taken such sentiments to heart in the same way as they were to abide by so many of the wiser principles of the Father of Medicine. The familial sense of loyalty fostered among the physicians of the Greek island of Cos some 2000 years earlier would have blended neatly with the hereditary system of the Gaels. There would equally have been nothing inconsistent with the names mentioned in the Book of Deer and the Wardlaw MS belonging to medical men as well as landowners and local officials. As John Bannerman points out in *The Beatons*, seventh- and eighth-century Gaelic law tracts accorded physicians 'the privileges of nobles in virtue of their professional skills, and they maintained this position into the late medieval period in both Gaelic Scotland and Ireland'.

It may even be said that the appointments of Dr Alexander Macleod of Kilpheader (of whom more later in this chapter) as chamberlain to the Macleod and Macdonald chiefs was a nineteenth-century acknowledgment of an ancient tradition.

Nevertheless, as Bannerman's extensive research reveals and confirms, the blood-ties of the Beatons and other medical kindreds were the overriding factor in their professional networks, and their debt to Irish learning is comparable with that of the early Celtic church in Scotland. But just as the Celtic church appears to have derived inspiration for its splendidly illuminated manuscripts, of which the Book of Kells is the outstanding example, partly from the art and craftsmanship of the Picts, so the medieval medicine of the Scottish Gaels must surely have incorporated a number of the medical practices of their Highland forerunners.

Such was the reputation of these men – no woman is recorded as a professional physician in the medieval Highlands, though many would have pursued their roles as unofficial healers – that their access to patronage was virtually immune to the political and physical conflicts of the day. When the Lordship of the Isles was forfeited to the crown in 1493, patronage of the clan physicians continued; and the 1609 Statutes of Iona (see below) did not legislate against the traditional employment of doctors.

The Macdonald Lordship of the Isles had emerged from its roots in the Norse/Gaelic kingdom of Man and the Isles – which ended when Norway ceded the Western Isles to Scotland in 1266 – to form a potent dynasty which created stability in the Gaidhealtachd and deep suspicion in the Lowlands. Its bonds with Ireland, the Isle of Man, and the Lordship of Galloway further added to its political strength. As much Scandinavian as Celtic in its origin, it was to build on the latter cultural heritage to establish an assertively self-conscious, and self-confident, Gaelic society.

It patronised poets and lawyers, churchmen and musicians, histor-ians and genealogists, scribes and record-keepers, and physicians. All of these would have been as much prized for enhancing the overall prestige of the Lordship as for their individual skills. Unfortunately for the image, Lowland Scotland was unable to appreciate the beauties of Gaelic poetry, and the system of law and the histories were viewed as esoteric. In his seminal paper, 'Gaelic Learned Orders and Literati in Medieval Scotland',[4] Derick Thomson has some interesting remarks on the ecclesiastics and, in particular, on the Gaelic/Latin/Scots trilingual Dean of Lismore, James MacGregor (d. 1551), who appears to have been increasingly drawn to the Scots tradition. The *Book of the Dean of Lismore*, a collection of Gaelic poetry from *c*.1310 to *c*.1520, is notable for basing its Gaelic orthography on the contemporary spelling of Scots. Thomson says, although recent research appears to qualify his suggestion: 'I think many Argyllshire clerics of his day must have looked askance at the Dean's system, if they knew of it, and regarded him with disfavour as a Scotticised Perthshire innovator.'

In a similar manner Lowland society came to view Gaelic ways as Celticised anachronisms. The power vacuum left by the suppression of the Lords of the Isles in 1493 resulted in a collapse of order and over a century of inter-clan turmoil from which developed a wary view of the Gaels as mere battle-happy and unlettered hillbillies. True enough, many chiefs did run what can be described only as protection rackets and they employed 'heavy men' as their agents. It was largely the activities of such men, a minority within wider Highland society, that gave rise to unfavourable opinions of the Gaels as a whole.

In his *History of Greater Britain*, published in 1521, the Berwickshire-born Scots historian, John Major (or Mair), divided his fellow countrymen not so much into Highlanders and Lowlanders as into 'Wild Scots' and 'Householding Scots'. 'One half of Scotland speaks Irish, and these as well as the Islanders we reckon to belong to the Wild Scots,' he wrote. His fellow Lowlanders were described as 'quiet and civil-living people' who led a 'decent and reasonable life', whereas the Highlanders were seen as 'following their own worthless and savage chief in all evil courses sooner than they would pursue an honest industry'. Major was born in 1470 when the Lordship of the Isles still flourished. Had he cared to look more closely behind the developing chaos following its suppression, he would have discovered a society which respected the arts and learning, where poets were well rewarded and even scribes and record-keepers had been granted lands in appreciation of their skills.

The power-centre of the Lordship was a small island in Loch

Finlaggan in Islay where the ruins of its council chamber still stand. There, each new lord was installed after the fashion of the ancient kings of Dalriada. Clothed in white and stepping into a footmark carved in a seven-foot square stone, the Macdonald rulers were given a white rod and a sword symbolising power and protection. Meetings were held at a huge stone table which seated the lord himself and the fourteen supreme councillors of the Isles. It is said that the Scots Court of Session, established in 1532 and known as the 'auld fifteen', was modelled on the Finlaggan procedure. Far from being lawless – except to those who would conquer it – Highland society of those times was highly, even rigidly, structured.

So innate was its regard for learning and education, that in all the tribulations that followed its collapse the people were to retain that respect for the cultivation of the mind to the extent that even the dire material poverty of the nineteenth century continued to produce many gifted people from the humblest of origins. Many sacrifices were made by needy families in order to provide higher education for the brighter children and, where that proved impossible, many formally unqualified people remained to enrich their communities with the deftness of their minds.

Unlike the occupations of the other learned orders, the practice of medicine transcended cultural and linguistic distinctions. As well as support from the clan chiefs who provided lands and funded their formal education, Highland physicians found prestigious patronage at the Scottish court.

The earliest known of these medieval Gaelic-speaking medical men practising in Scotland was Patrick MacBeth, chief physician and surgeon to Robert I (the Bruce). Patrick's son, Gilbert, was physician to David II and while that king was imprisoned in England between 1346 and 1357 Gilbert's name is recorded on documents allowing him safe-conduct to visit Scotland on the king's behalf. According to tradition, every king from Robert I to James VI employed a Beaton doctor. Bannerman writes:

This can certainly be confirmed for Robert I and David II and probably also for every king of Scots up to and including James IV. What can be demonstrated conclusively is that in every reign from that of Robert I to Charles I there were Beaton doctors, often more than one at any given time, on the payroll of the crown . . . It is noteworthy that a Lowland Scot, Hector Boece, describing in general terms the Gaelic learned orders in his Scottorum Historiae published for King James V in 1527 and translated into Scots by John Bellenden c. 1533, specifically singles out the profession of medicine, stating that "thay . . . are richt excellent in it".[5]

Other Gaelic-speaking medical men also achieved high office. Duncan Omey, who came of a scholarly family from Kintyre, was made principal surgeon to James V in 1526, and a Donegal doctor Niall Ó Glacáin, author of Tractatus de Peste (1629), was appointed physician to the King of France. But respect was given not only to the medical knowledge of the official Highland doctors. Many otherwise untutored Gaels gained a popular reputation for their skill in dissolving stones in the bladder and in remedial bleeding as well as for general healing knowledge.

Alongside, and in many ways oblivious of, the officially documented genealogies and histories of the official doctors, the people wove stories which, if largely apocryphal, show the esteem in which they were held and how very much an integral part they were of clan society. They were even endowed with the prestige of a 'creation myth' telling how they originally came by their medical knowledge and wisdom, the ultimate sanction of a place in the melting-pot of legend.

There are two main versions of this story, one emanating from Islay, the other from Sutherland. The latter account tells how, once long ago, Fearchar, a cattle drover from the north was at a market stance in the Lowlands when he was warmly greeted by a strange gentleman who inquired where he had come by his fine hazel stock.

'In Glen Golly in the Reay country,' replied Fearchar. 'Would you know the tree from which it was cut?' asked the stranger. 'Indeed, yes, if I were near it,' said the drover.

'I will give you a rich reward if you go to that tree and see whether there is a serpent's hole beneath it. If there is, wait a while and you will see six serpents coming out. Do not molest them, but wait until they return, when you will see a white serpent come in last. Catch this white serpent, bring it to me and a rich reward is yours.'

Judging that the man would be as good as his word, Fearchar agreed to the strange request. On his return home he went to the tree and saw the serpents exactly as the stranger had foretold. When he next met up with the stranger he produced the white serpent carefully sealed in a bottle. The gentleman was delighted and, to Fearchar's amazement, unstopped the bottle and shook the adder into a pot that was simmering on a fire at the roadside.

'I have to go away for a short while,' said the stranger. 'Mind you keep your eye on the pot till I return, and watch that it doesn't boil over.'

The man was not long gone, when the liquid began to boil. However the drover tried to dampen the fire, the boiling continued furiously until it looked set to lift the iron lid off altogether. As Fearchar tried to press the lid back down he burned one of his fingers and instinctively thrust it in his mouth.

> Lo and behold! the eyes of his understanding were opened, and he was made wise unto the healing of every ache and pain which ever befell mortal man. His host at last returned, and the first thing he did was to take off the pot lid, dip his finger in the bree and put it in his mouth. 'Oh,' he said, turning to Fearchar, 'this is of no good now. You did not as I told you, and hence no reward will I give.' It could not be undone or altered now.[6]

In his new wisdom, Fearchar was aware he now had a gift more precious than gold, and on his way home he healed all the sick people he met with. One day he neared a castle where the king was in agonies and unable to walk from a badly infected leg. Nothing the king's physicians did relieved or healed the pain. Hearing of this, Fearchar went to the gate and cried in Gaelic: '*A' bhiast-dubh air a' chnàmh gheal!*' ('The black beetle on the white bone!')

The king, hearing the shout, asked for the traveller to be brought to him. 'Are you a doctor?' asked the king. 'Indeed I am, sir,' replied Fearchar. 'If you heal me,' declared the king, 'I will give you what you ask, even to the half of my kingdom.'

Fearchar then revealed that instead of trying to cure him, the court physicians, for some political reason, had been keeping the king's ulcer open by setting beetles to gnaw at the flesh. After a proper poultice had been applied and the leg was healed, the grateful king inquired as to Fearchar's fee.

'The fee', said Fearchar Lighiche (Farquhar the Leech) as he was to be known from then on, 'is every island in the sea between Stoer Head in Assynt and the Red point in Orkney.' 'Granted,' said the king, 'along with much land in your own country besides.'

Here the legend, which has elements in common with Norse and Irish folk tales, merges with historical record. A royal charter[7] dated 4 September 1379 confirms a grant of the lands of Melness and Hope in north Sutherland by Robert II and his illegitimate son, Alexander Stewart (the Wolf of Badenoch), to 'Ffercado medico nostro' (Fearchar our physician). In a further charter, dated 31 December 1386, Robert II grants 'our esteemed and faithful leech Fearchar' a number of islands from Stoer Point in Assynt to Armadale on the north coast 'for his service done and to be done to us'. In the original charter the first of these islands is called Jura but it is not the island known as Jura today. In Robert II's time it was also the name of the one in Eddrachillis Bay now known as Oldaney.[8] In 1511 the lands of Melness and Hope were resigned by a descendant of Fearchar to the chiefs of the Mackays. The title to the islands must have been resigned somewhat earlier, as in 1504 they were gifted to Aodh Mackay by James IV.

Some of this branch of the Beatons may have remained in the north as physicians to the Mackay chiefs, but oral tradition has it that the main line of Fearchar's descendants became, under the name of Beaton, hereditary physicians to the Munros of Foulis, in Easter Ross. The Munro Writs record the names of Beaton doctors from the early sixteenth century onwards, although they claimed to have held lands in the area at least as far back as the thirteenth century.

In the west and in the isles, numerous branches of the Beatons flourished alongside other hereditary medical kindreds such as the O'Conachers (or MacConachers) of Lorn, the Macphails of Muckairn, a family of Macleans in Skye, the MacLachlans of Craiginterve, the MacMurchie physicians of Islay and the Clann MhicDhuinnshléibhe (Livingstones). One of the most prestigious of all these families was the Beatons of Balinaby in Islay, physicians to the Macdonald Lords of the Isles. Along with the leading Mull physicians they attracted the title *Ollamh*, whose meaning is on a par with 'professor'.

When in 1609 the Statutes of Iona required the chiefs of the Isles to swear allegiance to the crown, a number of restrictions and criteria were imposed. The stipulations included: that the heirs of men of substance (i.e. those who owned sixty or more cattle) were to be educated in the south 'sufficientlie to speik, reid, and wryte Inglische'; the carrying of firearms was to be prohibited; church ministers were to be planted in parishes and 'reverentlie obeyit'; and bards, along with vagabonds and jugglers, were to be banished. Such measures were part of an attempt to bring the isles and western seaboard into line with the other Gaelic-speaking areas which had become progressively assimilated into the legislative mainstream of Scotland.

Far from being brought under any restrictions – except, presumably, those relating to the English education of heirs – Fergus Beaton, for one, was confirmed in his landholdings of Balinaby and Oa in Islay, and in his family's role as chief physician to the Isles. In 1629 the lands passed into the ownership of the Campbells and the original house at Balinaby was completely destroyed by fire in 1933; however, an old walled garden behind the present farmhouse may yet provide fruitful research for archaeo-botanists.

What these professional men gave to Highland medicine was theory, philosophy, ethics and a system based mainly on Greek, Islamic, and Continental sources. Along with these they combined many traditional methods and remedies. Just how much native practice pervaded their day-to-day procedures, it remains hard to say. Of the twenty-nine surviving Gaelic medical manuscripts of the period only a fraction of the text has been translated. It might be argued that medical texts as such are not necessarily an accurate guide to actual practice, since individual doctors would have their own routines and ideas and might have been restricted in the material remedies available to them.

However, the manuscripts are not only obviously working manuals with jottings in the margins and signs of contemporary wear and tear, but also collections of earlier, mainly classical and Arabic, writings which arguably reflect the individual preferences of the compilers.

As to where the official medicine of the Highlands diverges from the orthodox teaching of medieval Europe, Ronald Black, cataloguer of Gaelic manuscripts in the National Library of Scotland, says:

> Jottings in the margins and blank spaces of manuscripts tend to reveal the physician meeting the day-to-day realities of reassuring patients (aphorisms) and providing them with the weapons they sought for their battles against disease, aging, sterility, injury and death (charms). In medical terms none of this is unique among European traditions; what is distinctive is the apparent convergence of interests between doctor and patient . . . The language of the texts is not secret jargon, but a simple Early Modern Gaelic comprehensible everywhere from Melness to Munster. One has the impression that the Beatons were doctors who listened to their patients as well as talking to them. Certainly no other scribal tradition in European palaeography makes so free with marginalia, and these, along with condition, provide clues as to the extent to which texts were used.[9]

These medical manuscripts may have survived in such a quantity partly because of the very nature of the books and the fact that they were compiled for and circulated within a small circle of family and professional connections. The cost of copying a Gaelic version of Bernard of Gordon's great fourteenth-century medical work, the *Lilium Medicinae*, was, according to the Revd Donald MacQueen (1740–85) of Kilmuir in Skye, sixty milk cows. 'The copy possessed by Farchar Beaton of Husabost five generations ago,' MacQueen noted, '. . . was of such value in his estimation that when he trusted himself to a boat, in passing an arm of the sea, to attend any patient at Dunvegan, the seat of MacLeod, he sent his servant by land, for the greater security, with the *Lilium Medicinae*.'[10]

The *Aphorisms* of Hippocrates is the most popular single text cited in the Gaelic medical manuscripts, followed by constant quoting from other Hippocratic works with their emphasis on the importance of diagnosis and clinical observation. From Islamic medicine the Gaelic doctors culled pharmacology, dermatology, astrology and alchemy. While the latter two subjects were viewed askance by later practitioners of 'rational' medicine, it should be remembered that they were the forerunners of scientific astronomy and chemistry. The *Aphorisms* of Johannnes Damascenus (777–857) come second in popularity, and there are frequent references to other Arabian works such as those of Isaac Israeli[11] (d.893), whose writings on fevers, diet and urine were standard medical texts in Europe for many centuries, and Avicenna (980–1037), the Persian who was to become the most famous of the Arab physicians. Much of the ethos derives or is directly quoted from the philosophy of Aristotle.

The education of Highland physicians at the leading Continental centres of medical learning is a strong influence on the Gaelic texts. Virtually from their foundation, the early universities, such as Paris (1110) and Bologna (1158), had, alongside the other two principal faculties of theology and law, taught medicine (after a fashion and based largely on the theory contained in classical texts), but a distinctive Continental form of medicine had already begun to develop at the notable medical school of Salerno, founded in c.850 near the Benedictine monastery of Monte Cassino just south of Naples. For its time Salerno was undoubtedly far-seeing, broad-minded and innovative, not least in that it was a rare lay institution of learning. Most unusually, outside of certain convents which fostered such intellects as that of St Hildegard of Bingen (1098–1179), it encouraged women both as students and teachers, the most famous of whom was Trotula – remembered in English nursery rhyme as 'Dame Trot' – who wrote an influential book on obstetrics in about 1050.

Although, so far as is known, Highland women were not formally educated in the official medicine of the time, the advanced ideals of Salerno, which disregarded restrictions of colour, creed and class, permeate Gaelic medical writings. Its most renowned text, the *Regimen Sanitatum Saliternae*, with its accent on the maintenance of health and prevention of sickness by a moderate way of life and attention to diet and exercise, is reflected in the *Regimen Sanitatis* (Rule of Health) compiled by John Beaton of Islay (fl. 1563).

This Rule of Health, the manuscript of which is in the British Library in London, was published in a rather ungainly and flawed English translation by Dr Hugh Cameron Gillies in 1911 but, for the time being, it remains the only fully translated medieval Scottish Gaelic medical work. (The Irish Texts Society's edition of a Gaelic translation of John of Gaddesden's *Rosa Anglica* (c.1314) is a more useful English version of a comparable work.) Despite its flaws, Gillies' work on the manuscript and his other writings remain a worthy attempt to raise the status of, and serious interest in, Gaelic medicine. Had he been pursuing his interests today he would have had the benefit of further generations of Gaelic scholarship at his disposal.

However unwieldy in translation, the Gaelic Regimen Sanitatis throws interesting light on the health-conscious Highlander of the Middle Ages, for the concern with preventing disease and the pursuit of a sensible way of life parallel modern society's preoccupations. The three main principles of health with which the book begins guide the thinking throughout: the understanding and conservation of what makes for a healthy mind and body, the importance of noting the early signs of a breakdown in health and the means of preventing it, and the healing of the sick. One of the most significant aspects of the Gaelic doctors' beliefs was that health is maintained largely through applying common sense and, if somewhat sweepingly, that illness is chiefly caused by lack of it.

After rising in the morning the Gael was advised to stretch his arms and chest, have a good clean spit and rub dust and sweat from the skin. Hair was to be combed, hands and face washed *and* the teeth cleaned. After a prayer, some good exercise and walking in 'high clean places' was to be undertaken before breakfast.

Stringent advice on diet included guidance on cooking that took the then scientifically unidentified risks of salmonella poisoning into account:

> It should be known also that great injury is caused by the raw things such as oysters, and the things half raw as are the birds that are badly roasted . . .

In recommending eggs and egg custard for invalids, the manuscript notes:

> . . . if they are got in an unclean vessel they are very easily fouled, and they are the more healthy if broken into water.

Advice to cook peas, beans and other pulses with a pinch of cumin in order to prevent embarrassing bouts of wind is a tip worth remembering. An invalid dish of the white heads of leeks, boiled, strained and mixed with milk of almonds sounds a delicacy. After blood-letting, convalescents were to have a light but vitamin-rich meal of kale, mallow, sage and parsley. In summer this was varied with the addition of borage, bugloss, violets, spinach, lettuce, the tops of fennel and other herbs.

When it came to drinking habits, the counselling was complex. Quoting Avicenna on wine-drinking, the Beaton doctor cautions: '[It] is like putting fire upon the head of fire on weakly wood if given to youths.' But he also questions some orthodox advice, as when Avicenna was assumed to be warning against taking wine with food. This, says the physician, surely cannot mean no wine with a meal, but that wine should not be taken in the same mouthful as food.

Drink taken in moderation was advocated, over-indulging, as in anything, severely frowned upon. A paean to whisky in a manuscript held in the National Library of Scotland and assembled largely in the first half of the seventeenth century by several Mull Beatons, can rarely have been equalled:

> . . . it will heal wounds and it will brighten brass, and it will help those suffering from fistula and round cancer, and if it be given to epileptics in their drink it will help them, and it will cure every gripe or colic caused by cold or paralysis, and it will sharpen the wits, and it will make you remember the things you have forgotten, and it will make the sad man into a happy man, and it will preserve youth for everybody, and it will remove the impurities of the night, and it will soothe and cure those who suffer from salty phlegm, and it will dispel toothache and remove putrid matter from the nose and from the roots of the teeth and from the jaw, and it will burst the quinsy, that is imposthumes of the throat . . . and it will most marvellously help . . . the melancholia and it will be adequate for sciatica and it will cure the dropsy that is caused by cold and it will help the colic fever and it will reduce poison and throat disease and deafness of the ears, and should a man suffering from leprosy drink it, it will get no worse than it is, and it will help women to conceive, and it will shift the catarrh if the person keeps it in his mouth, and it will help headache if the head is rubbed with it, and it will help trembling limbs . . . and it is gentler than water of roses, and it floats on oil and on every mixture of wine and water if poured on them . . . and it makes good wine out of stale wine and strong wine out of weak wine and very good wine out of good wine . . .[12]

It is worth noting here that the late medieval medicinal use of whisky, as recommended in the Beaton manuscripts, was to drink only a small amount mixed with a little meal or milk. The spirit probably derived a lot of its virtues from the aromatic herbs then used for flavouring and which included fennel, thyme, mint, anise, juniper and cranberries.

Alongside a wealth of native materials, the manuscripts list a fair assortment of exotic ones. The book officially catalogued Advocates Manuscript 72.2.10 was compiled by Aonghas mac Fhearchair mhic Aonghais, one of the Husabost (Skye) line who were the most prolific writers of Gaelic medical works, and its prescriptions give a wide use of materia. Among them Aonghas lists water melon, cashew, tamarind, lapis lazuli, senna, myrrh, nutmeg, Spanish flies (the cantharides beetle), ginger, camphor, coriander, calcined elephant-bone, Persian gum, aloes, cassia and opium.[13]

The more exotic drugs and plant materials probably found their way into the Highlands by the same route, from the Mediterranean via (usually) Ireland, used by the chiefs to import their French wines, Spanish swords, and silks. There is evidence of Irish trade with the Near East from at least the sixth century onwards and the Scandinavians, too, had strong eastern links from early times. The north and west of Scotland could call on both its Irish and Norse links and, no doubt, these were a strengthening factor in the physicians' belief in and use of Arabian remedies in addition to native ones.

The largest Gaelic manuscript was copied in 1612 by Angus, son of Farquhar Beaton of Husabost in Skye, from a manuscript already in the possession of the MacConachers of Ardoran, and, aside from its other content, is interesting for Beaton's name being written at least twice (on pages 302 and 401) in a code which, on examination, turns out to be based on the Ogham alphabet of the earlier Gaels and Picts.

On page 302, for example, is written (originally in Gaelic): 'I am **bhdlnqhfts mbhc fscbhrcbhnqr** – which deciphered, means Aonghus Mac Fearcair.' Each vowel is represented by a pair of consonants – bh = a, nq = i, sc = e ft = u dl = o – which in turn correspond with pairs of 'mirror-image' strokes in the Ogham inscriptions on Pictish symbol stones. For example the Ogham stroke for **B** is / (above the line) and for **H** \ (below the line), where **A** equals one stroke above and below; similarly **D** \\ is (above the line), and **L** is // (below the line), where **O** is two strokes above and below. Each of Angus's codes for a vowel similarly suggest an Ogham base.

It is tempting to wonder whether a closer perusal of what other occasional codes may exist in the medieval texts might help to throw a modicum of light on the abiding mystery of the meaning of Pictish Oghams. The Celtic druids were traditionally said to enjoy indulging in word-games and riddles. Perhaps as well as something of their bardic and healing lore, other aspects of their knowledge were passed down to the Gaelic learned orders of later times.

For reasons which remain a mystery but may not be unrelated to the fact that its liberalism stretched, undesirably in the view of the church, to including Jewish medicine and culture in the curriculum, Salerno declined in influence and the torch of medical learning passed to other centres. In the thirteenth and fourteenth centuries the leading university medical school became that of Montpellier in the South of France.

It was there that one of the Beaton physicians is said to have translated the *Lilium Medicinae* of Bernard de Gordon (installed as Professor of Medicine at Montpellier in 1285) at some time in the sixteenth century. Montpellier continued to attract Scottish medical students, both Highland and Lowland, until Leiden, after Bologna and Padua, overtook it in popularity and status in the seventeenth century. On a visit to Leiden a few years ago I was able to examine the records of the Scottish medical graduates and post-graduates of the period among whom were the names of several Beatons and also that of the Skyeman Martin Martin who entered the university there in the 1710. After Leiden, Edinburgh was to become the leading centre of medical teaching but by that time the distinctive clan patronage of physicians was already a matter of history.

During the 400 years in which the Gaelic medical kindreds flourished, European medicine was still dominated by diagnosis and treatment through the 'doctrine of humours' which had its origins in the fifth-century BC theory of Empedocles that all matter consisted of four elements: earth, air, fire and water. To this Anaxagoras (500–428 BC) and Aristotle (384–322 BC) had added the four qualities of all matter, hot, cold, dry and wet. Disease came to be regarded as an imbalance of the humours: blood, phlegm, yellow bile and black bile which respectively controlled sanguine, phlegmatic, choleric and melancholic temperaments. It was believed that disorders could best be corrected by administering remedies judged to embody the regulating 'quality'. All of these and many other mainstream medieval ideas are followed in the Gaelic 'official' tradition. In line with establishment thinking of the time, the medical investigations of da Vinci and Vesalius are ignored (except for one reference to the latter in an Irish text) in favour of a lingering trust in the theories of the second-century Graeco-Roman physician Galen.

The most popular European texts in the manuscripts are a version of *Liber de Simplici Medicina, dictus Circa Instans*, a pharmacopoeia compiled in *c.* 1150 at Salerno from earlier sources, and de Gordon's *Lilium Medicinae*, already mentioned. The Gaelic version of *Circa Instans* which was compiled at Montpellier in 1415 by an Irishman, Tadhg Ó Cuinn, survives in at least fifteen copies, and is currently being studied by scholars in Ireland and Scotland. Prognosis was by uroscopy and astrology, and both of these receive considerable attention in the manuscripts. The Highland doctors' skill in making astute deductions from the observation and testing of urine samples was legendary. One popular tale recounted how a king of Scots was ill and a Beaton was summoned from the Highlands. Jealous and cunning court physicians replaced the king's specimen with cow's urine, but the *Ollamh* outmatched them. Holding the glass phial up to the light, he solemnly declared: 'If you gentlemen open up His Majesty, you will find him in calf!'

This somewhat apocryphal story has an even more vivid counterpart in one told of the Mull *Ollamh*, Seumas Beaton, who was sent for by a gentleman at his wits' end with pain. The patient, a Maclean of Duart, was lying sick at Aros Castle, in Mull, prostrate with a painful illness that two eminent physicians brought in from the mainland had been treating to no avail. Seumas, the island doctor from Pennycross, asked to see Maclean alone, swiftly diagnosed the problem and knew the only cure would be some sudden, violent exertion of the lungs. But how to bring this about in such a weakened patient?

In front of the amazed, and doubtless horrified, Maclean, the *Ollamh Muileach* grabbed the shovel by the hearth, took down his breeches and proceeded to fill it with his own excrement which he then roasted over the fire until it was dry enough to be powdered. The unlikely preparation was then wrapped in paper and placed half-opened on the bedside table. All this was done in silence. Giving no instructions to the by now speechless Maclean, Beaton put a cautioning finger to his lips and left, promising to return the next day.

With the country leech out of the way, the city doctors rushed back to the sickroom (at whose door they had been listening to no advantage). Pompous, but eager to learn what had happened, they threw questions at the patient who merely waved weakly at the parcel of brown powder and murmured that Beaton had given no advice.

Inquisitively, the doctors poked and smelled the powder but could make nothing of it. Well, it seemed harmless enough. Together they took up good-sized pinches of the stuff and tasted and swallowed their country colleague's offering. It was too much, even for the enfeebled Maclean who just burst out laughing till he rocked with a force he did not know was left in him. It did the trick. The ulcer burst, he vomited up a quantity of foul matter and was set for a cure. A few days later Maclean was out hunting with the best of them again – and vowing to employ no more 'fashionable' doctors – while the

Ollamh was praised throughout the area as a man of great shrewdness and skill.

Bleeding, for the relief of certain illnesses and for the maintenance of health, was a common feature of medicine down to the nineteenth century and often caused more harm than good. It is to the credit of the Highland doctors that they recognised the drawbacks. 'Too frequent bloodletting', they note in their Rule of Health, 'causes apoplexy . . . [and] the practice of bloodletting more greatly weakens the vitality than all other practices.' Generally they seem to have followed the advice of Damascenus who recommended a maximum of four bleedings a year for the young, three after the age of forty, once a year after sixty and none at all after seventy.

The high reputation of Gaelic medicine rested mainly on its adherence to common sense, the use of simples, and the encouragement given to healthy ways of living by the medical men. The doctors even appear to have had a code of practice rooted in the old Gaelic system of concern for welfare, judging by a compilation of miscellaneous writings by Malcolm Beaton of Mull (fl. 1600) which contains a commentary on the Brehon Law of sick-maintenance.

The split and subsequent rivalries between physicians and barber-surgeons that occurred elsewhere did not afflict medical practice in the Highlands where the doctors had a good reputation in surgery. By the end of the seventeenth century the town of Glasgow was officially appointing Highland surgeons such as Iomhar MacNeill and Duncan Campbell for their particular skill in performing lithotomies.

In about 1550 it was written of the Balinaby doctors:

> Clann Mhic Beathadh, a gnáth grinn,
> Luchd snoidhe chnámh agus chuislenn.
> (The MacBeaths, accurate in their practice,
> Carvers of bones and arteries.)

Light instructional verses attributed to the doctors themselves include:

> Bi gu subhach geanmnaidh
> Moch-thràthach as t-samhradh,
> Bi gu curraiceach brògach
> Brochanach sa gheamhradh.
> (In summertime be cheerful, chaste
> And early out of bed,
> In winter be well capped, well shod,
> And well on porridge fed.)

And there was this advice for an old man from the Ollamh Ìleach:

> Cóinneach do 'thaigh,
> Crìonach a chonnadh;
> Blàth on bhoine,
> Teth on teine.
> (Moss for his house,
> Brushwood his fuel;
> Warm from the cow,
> Hot from the fire.)

Although they owned books which contained spells and exotic Arabian cures, there seems to be no evidence that the official physicians, who went from family to family, and place to place, healing high and low, were ever suspected of sorcery. Again, this may result from their reputation for common sense, however strange some remedies of the time may seem today. No affliction was too small for their attention and then as now people were as concerned with their appearance as with their general state of health. One prescription for the treatment of grey hair, curiously believed to be caused by 'phlegmatic humours of poor quality arising from the stomach', was to employ remedies for clearing phlegm.

Since 'cures' for baldness continue to be weird and wonderful, the following advice may intrigue the desperate, though somehow one cannot help suspecting a measure of knowing humour on the part of the healer who wrote this:

Fill an earthenware pippin with mice; stop the mouth of the pippin with a lump of clay and bury the whole beside a fire but do not let great heat of the fire reach it. So leave it for a year and then take out the contents of the pippin – being very careful that the one who handles this matter shall wear gloves, because if he does not, hair will come sprouting out of his finger-tips – and this, after further preparation, if applied to the head will cause hair to grow.[14]

In a letter dated Dunvegan, 5 March 1823, and addressed to a supervisor of excise in Edinburgh, John Kelly writes:

The next [story] is that of Farquaar [sic] Bethune called in Gaelic Farquhar Leich which signifies the curer of every kind of diseases, and which knowledge he received from a book printed in red which had descended in heritable succession and is now in the possession of Kenneth Bethune . . . in Glendale, and which they contain both secret and sacred; what instructions are contained therein are descriptive of the virtues of certain herbs in particular which he denied having any equal, nor being produced by any other country by Skye, it has been examined by Botanists from London and elsewhere and its non-affinity to any other confirmed. He was gifted with prophecy, and held conf—[?conference] with the Brutal [natural] creation in that was quite a prodigy. This is only an outline of him.'[15]

One traditional story, however, shows one of the doctors in a decidedly bad light and, if true, may derive from one of many contemporary squabbles over rights to certain landholdings. Maclean of Aros, feeling slighted by a MacGillivray of Glencannell, drew his sword and took off the upper part of MacGillivray's skull. However, the latter's attendants took him home and called on the *Ollamh Muileach* to heal him. It was no easy matter, for the exposed brain was covered only by a thin membrane, but the Mull doctor was skilled and MacGillivray made good progress.

Hearing that the patient would soon be on his feet, Maclean told the doctor, 'You must kill him.' 'Certainly not,' replied the *Ollamh*. 'He never did me any harm.'

'If you don't kill him, I'll kill you,' said Maclean. 'My business is to heal men, not kill them,' insisted the doctor. 'If you kill him,' said Maclean, 'I'll give you the lands of Pennycross.'

The temptation was too great and the doctor insisted on being given the title to the lands there and then. On his way to see MacGillivray he picked a stalk of ryegrass and carried it with him. At the house the grateful patient declared that he was virtually mended. But the doctor insisted on removing the dressing and inspecting the wound, whereupon he began rubbing the membrane with the grass stalk until he made a hole in it.

MacGillivray understood perfectly what was happening and drew his sword to strike the devious doctor but the latter escaped while the effort caused the patient to fall and die. Maclean took over MacGillivray's lands and the Mull Doctor those of Pennycross.

The stories attached to a physician named Niall Òg are of a happier nature and portray him as a virtual miracle-worker. On one occasion he is said to have met a funeral party and proved that the 'corpse' was still alive. However, the mourners persisted in believing that the man had really died and he was restored only through Niall's wondrous powers.

Some years after his own death he appeared in a dream to the dying wife of a Clanranald chief in Uist. In despair that the very best doctors of the day had been unable either to diagnose her illness or provide any relief, she cried out to her nurses: 'Oh, I wish Niall Òg were here, he would know what to do.' Not long after, she fell into a deep sleep and dreamed that Niall Òg was standing by her bed giving her clear instructions. A boat was to be sent to Skye immediately and a rare plant that grew by a burn at the back of Healaval Mòr was to be brought back. Niall promised that from the very first drink of an infusion made from its leaves she would be on the way to recovery. The instructions were carried out and Lady Clanranald went on to live a healthy life for many years.

These traditional stories are not just idle entertainments, but evidence of the people's awareness of the doctors' skills. Even the grim tale told of how the Mull doctor acquired his lands does not question his expertise. The physicians' manuscripts are now impenetrable to all but a handful of Gaelic scholars, and their herb gardens gone – though the site at Pennycross is still remembered – but they live on vividly in folklore and, in the Gaelic way of things, the interests of their descendants.

Alexander Carmichael, the great collector of Gaelic folklore, was a friend of *Iain mac Fhearchair mhic Iain mhic Nèill Dotair*, John son of Farquhar son of John son of Doctor Neil, of Aird nan Laogh in South Uist, who died in 1881 at the age of ninety-two, and said of him that while he was a shepherd by occupation, he was a botanist by instinct, 'one of nature's scientists and nature's gentlemen'.

> He knew Gaelic only, and he knew no letters, but probably he knew more about plants and plant habitats and characteristics than any other man in Scotland. He lived in close communion with Nature, and loved plants as he loved his children – with a warm abiding love which no poverty could cool and no age could dim.

A by no means rare instance of the Beaton talents being handed down in the female line is given in a reminiscence by Dr Norman Maclean in 1945:

> Chirsty never claimed that her gift of healing was of her own merits. One day, when I was between ten and eleven years of age, I was sent in great haste to Chirsty to get some medicine for old Granny, who lived . . . beyond the hill wall. Granny had a violent attack of palpitation, and she had great faith in Chirsty's medicine. So my mother sent me running that mile and a half to the corner of the bay, and there I told Chirsty my errand. She at once set me on a chair

beside the fire while she quickly got the herbs she wanted and set them to boil on the fire. And while the pan tarried before boiling, Chirsty talked.

'How did you learn all your healing knowledge?' I asked shyly.

'I learned it from my grandfather,' she replied. 'My mother was a daughter of the last of the Bethunes, who for hundreds of years were the physicians of the Lord of the Isles. When I was a girl I spent much time with my grandfather, and he taught me the healing powers of the different herbs.'[16]

Mary Montgomery of Roag near Dunvegan, mother of the Gaelic poets Catriona and Morag Montgomery, was born a Beaton and remembered several interesting old cures for me in the 1970s. The tradition continues here and there in the present young generation. Helen Lindsay of Dunbeath in Caithness is the granddaughter of William Bethune, a repository of much of his ancestors' lore, who died in 1992 at the age of ninety-three. While still a schoolgirl at Wick in 1985 she won the Wendy Wood Award for a history project on Dunbeath and in the following year the Dunbeath Preservation Trust published her work, which includes local healing lore, in a small booklet.[17] Helen, now with a degree in chemical engineering, is working on pollution control in the oil industry – a worthy echo of John the Uist shepherd's care for nature.

Chronologically, the story of Alexander Macleod, the *Dotair Bàn*, and his family should find a place in a later chapter, but in so many other aspects they form one of the threads of Highland healing that link the more remote ethos and kindred system of the medieval physicians with more recent medical practice.

Alexander Macleod of Kilpheadar (or Kilphedder), North Uist[18], was a Hebridean-born Edinburgh-trained general practitioner in the islands between 1808-54.[19] So popular was he with his patients that he was widely and affectionately known to all by his by-name of *An Dotair Bàn*, and his ways and family background are a strong echo of the medical dynasties of the Middle Ages.

The *Dotair Bàn*'s family held much the same status as the medieval doctors, intermarrying with the indigenous upper classes of Highland society, being middle-ranking landowners, and benefiting from a university education as well as retaining respect for their native traditions and learning. They, like their forerunners in the medieval learned kindreds, represented an educated, often well-travelled, professional Gaelic middle-class forgotten in a popular image of Highland history that prefers to focus on aristocrats and peasants.

Alexander's father, Murdoch (*Murchadh*), was one of the Macleods of Rigg, a cadet branch of the Raasay Macleods who held land near Scorrybreck in Skye. As a young man Murdoch qualified as a surgeon-apothecary, probably in Edinburgh, and set out for the American colonies where he ran an apothecary shop in Cross Creek, North Carolina. Medicine was already in his blood. A Dr Murdoch Macleod of Raasay, attended the Jacobite army at Culloden in 1746, where he received a bullet wound from which he recovered sufficiently to help Charles Edward Stuart in his flight from Scotland. This Macleod set up a practice in Portree and was to have a son who fought with Nelson at Trafalgar. The Cross Creek apothecary was to follow the family tradition.

When the American War of Independence broke out in 1775, Murdoch joined the army as a surgeon, though unlike his namesake he tended not rebel but British government troops. He was taken prisoner but later returned to the Highlands on the same ship as that much-applauded Jacobite heroine, Flora Macdonald. Murdoch settled in Kilpheader, North Uist, where Alexander was born in 1788. After qualifying in 1808 the man who was to become known as *An Dotair Bàn* succeeded his father in the North Uist practice and three of his four brothers also entered medicine.

Murdoch junior practised in the West Indies, John became an army surgeon in England and Donald had a general practice in Hawick. One of Alexander's grandsons made a career in the army medical school in the south of England and another, Colonel Kenneth Macleod of the Indian Medical Service, was Professor of Surgery at Calcutta University.

Of the *Dotair Bàn* himself it was said it he was 'probably the most popular man who ever acted in that capacity in the Highlands'. Indeed, so many patients travelled to his North Uist surgery from other islands that his house at Balelone, Kilpheader, was likened to a hospital.

It was yet another grandson, Dr M (Murdoch?) D Macleod, medical superintendent of the East Riding Asylum, in Beverley, Yorkshire, at the end of the nineteenth century, who was to reveal to his colleagues in the Caledonian Medical Society one of the chief factors in the *Dotair Bàn*'s success story. The grandson related:

> He had a great reputation, not only in the islands, but practically in the whole shire, as a successful physician; much of his success was attributed by the natives to his use of the herbs growing locally as remedies. In this way he intensified the potency of his remedy (the therapeutic properties of which were well known to him) by working on the emotions of his patients. Many of the indigenous herbs have medicinal value – e.g. the gentians, the potentillas, the trefoils, the poppies – and infusions, tinctures and decoctions of them are, so far as they go, as useful as those manufactured from their tropical congeners which are richer in alkaloids.[20]

In 1854, Alexander Macleod was persuaded by Lord Macdonald to move to the practice of Strath and Sleat in Skye which also included the Knoydart area of the mainland. His first visit to Knoydart was made in April that same year. On his return at night from the urgent call to a shepherd's wife in a remote house reached only by a long walk over trackless moorland, he lost his way in the dark and fell to the bottom of a sixty-foot precipice. When his body was found two days later, the only relief was that he appeared to have died instantly. He was buried in Kilmuir, North Uist, and his loss was deeply mourned throughout the islands.

Such a man, from a professional family, dutiful and educated, yet at the same time in tune with his patients and steeped in the lore of his people, combining orthodox medicine with native herbal wisdom, was, in practice and outlook, a direct heir of the medieval clan doctors of Gaeldom. When the historian John Bannerman was in Grenitote, North Uist, in August 1983, he heard the story of the doctor, excrement and the burst ulcer told not of Seumas Beaton but of the admired and much-loved *Dotair Bàn*, recited during a house ceilidh. The only other change was that instead of a powder, the unlikely 'medicine' was made up into *pilichean*, 'pills'.

The Dr Murdoch Macleod of Raasay who tended the wounded at Culloden was one of many physicians employed by the Jacobite and Hanoverian armies. By 1746 the unique clan patronage of Highland medicine had disappeared and such names as MacConacher and Beaton do not figure among the lists of clan medical men on the battlefield. Notably, however, yet another new Highland dynasty of physicians, the Monros, who were to gain international fame over several generations, was represented in the '45 by Alexander Monro, by then Professor of Anatomy at the University of Edinburgh. Alexander was, like most of his clan, a Hanoverian, but interceded for his former students despite their allegiances and treated the wounded impartially. Again, and typically of the sad confusions of the strife in which the closest of blood-ties found themselves on opposing sides, a medically qualified Macleod of Talisker aligned himself with the government and a Dr John Monro tended Jacobites. The full story of the Highland military doctors is too long a one to be told in detail here.[21]

Although they always seem to have had a leaning to wider Gaelic scholarship, the physicians' interests in this direction were to blossom more fully in the years when their medical ones had declined. The Revd John Beaton (*c.* 1640–1715), minister of Kilninian in Mull 1670–1701, was the son of the last of the Mull *Ollamhan* and a valuable source of the Gaelic learning and lore collected by the Celtic scholar Edward Lhuyd (1660–1709). Christopher MacBeath compiled the greater part of the Black Book of Clanranald, a collection of history, genealogy and poems by the MacMhuirich bards and others in the early eighteenth century.

In his presidential address to the Caledonian Medical Society in 1904, George Mackay, a Fellow of the Royal College of Surgeons of Edinburgh, ended by pleading for the transcription and translation of the medieval Gaelic medical manuscripts:

> It is a service which we ought to render to our country, and by its accomplishment we should rear a memorial to the men from whom we are proud to trace our professional descent.

Ninety years further on, Mackay's plea is only just beginning to be heeded, and most Scots remain unaware of the extraordinary wealth of medical art and science that existed in the 'wild' Highlands for some four centuries before the old culture was largely extinguished.

5

HIGHLAND MEDICINE AND THE ENLIGHTENMENT

The decline of the old clan patronage structure of medicine together with the general breaking down of the traditional social order turned the aspirations of the medical kindreds in other directions. Many of their sons were now to enter the church or teaching and those who remained loyal to their ancestral profession turned their sights to the Lowlands and beyond, into a world of new political and cultural perspectives.

The 1707 Treaty of Union did not only terminate an independent parliament. The nobility and wealthy and influential patrons looked to the south and its ways, the Lowland Scots language became marginalised by polite society, and there were all the signs of a culture breaking apart. From this unlikely setting was to evolve the splendid period in which Edinburgh became one of the leading intellectual centres of Europe. Partly it may not have been so much a paradox or a swansong, as a natural counteraction: the need to fill a vacuum. That this was met not only by unrest but by a fusion of the country's best minds under the banner of the Scottish Enlightenment is an enduring tribute to the essential genius of a people who wrought their learning in as tough a setting as that in which they tilled their fields. It can also be argued that that fruitful period for the arts and learning would have occurred without the catalyst of the Union, just as a similar flourishing occurred during the reign of James IV. From the point of view of the arts and sciences, the Union and the turmoil caused by the Jacobite uprisings can be seen as a hiatus between developments in the second half of the seventeenth century and those of a hundred years after. As William Ferguson has remarked: '. . . not a few old and familiar aspects of Scottish society . . . contributed to, and made possible, the dynamic movement known as the Enlightenment'.[1] The theological rigours of the Kirk, the philosophical bent of the law, the principles of education, all of which institutions were to remain independent of the English system, combined to hone a particularly tenacious and inquiring turn of mind with a penchant for debate and analysis.

Medicine was to flourish alongside philosophy, chemistry, litera-ture, painting and architecture, and if Edinburgh came more lately to the advances in medical practice and thinking that had begun in Europe decades earlier and were to reach a high point in the teaching of the great Hermann Boerhaave of Leiden (1688–1738), it was to rise to pre-eminence in that field by the second half of the eighteenth century.

The lure of Edinburgh, and later the other Scottish medical schools, as much as the local breakdown of the old order, was to prove irresistible to the men of the Highland tradition. Medical students who in earlier times had found their way from, say, Mull to Montpellier and home again, now found a better climate for advancement outwith their own society. The professional Gaelic tradition was conservative and becoming increasingly atrophied. Instead of infusing the new scientific ideas into their own tradition, the hereditary physicians blended into the wider scene. This might have opened opportunities for, as it were, new blood to practise medicine in the Highlands, but it was not to occur for many years. The chiefs and their families, increasingly alienated from the people, could afford the ministrations of southern doctors. The vast majority of people could not and they leaned more and more heavily on their old remedies.

Yet if the medicine of the hereditary physicians was beginning to look increasingly old-fashioned when measured against the new scien-ces, the even more ancient folk cures had begun to attract attention from what was to become the new heart of learning itself.

Robert Sibbald (1641–1722), who became the first Professor of Medicine at the University of Edinburgh in 1685, was a man of many parts, a geographer, antiquary, naturalist and prolific writer as well as a physician. He began the Physic Garden which was to become the Royal Botanic Garden and was one of the founders of the Royal College of Physicians of Edinburgh. Of a Fife landed family, he had a lifelong interest in all matters Scottish, stimulating other writers to follow his histories and area surveys of the country.

As a doctor he explored the relationship between poverty and disease with a sympathetic understanding of the poor and what might be done to better their condition. His interest in nature and the common people and his wariness of the complex pharmacopoeia of his time were to have a profound influence on Scottish medical thinking. Sibbald and his contemporary Archibald Pitcairne (1652–1713) were, in the seventeenth century, to sow the seeds of Scotland's eighteenth-century pre-eminence in medicine.

Most relevantly in a Highland context, Sibbald was the mentor of the intrepid and thoughtful Martin Martin, a Gaelic-speaking Skyeman, who, prompted by Sibbald's own interests, made an invaluable collection of the local remedies in the islands and in doing so learned to respect the ideas, values and wealth of native knowledge behind the traditional practices.

Examples of the numerous cures that Martin found throughout the islands are cited elsewhere in this book. Here it is worth looking closely at his preface where he writes:

> The inhabitants of these [western] islands . . . seem to be better versed in the Book of Nature, than many that have greater Opportunities of Improvement. This will appear plain and evident to the judicious Reader, upon a View of the successful Practice of the Islanders in the Preservation of their Health, above what the Generality of Mankind enjoys; and this is perform'd merely by Temperance, and the prudent use of Simples; which, as we are assured by repeated Experiments, fail not to remove the most stubborn Distempers, where the best

prepar'd Medicines have frequently no Success. This I relate not only from the Authority of many of the Inhabitants, who are Persons of great Integrity, but likewise from my own particular Observation. And thus with Celsus, they first make Experiments, and afterwards proceed to reason upon the Effects.[2]

The specific reference to the Greek writer is interesting. Though not a physician himself, Cornelius Celsus wrote an important work known in its Latin translation (the original Greek text having been lost) as *De Re Medicina* in *c.* AD 30. The collection of advice and theory is, like the later Gaelic medical works, derived mainly from the Hippocratic writings with their accent on the healing force of nature. Modern medicine somehow persists, formally at least, in calling this force the *vis medicatrix naturae,* as if, while having to recognise its undoubted existence, scientific embarrassment at anything so indefinable is mitigated by a Latin tag. The people whose cures Martin collected were more interested in necessities than theoretical niceties; they simply tried to hasten the healing *force* of nature by using the *produce* of nature. Martin continues:

Human Industry has of late advanc'd useful and experimental Philosophy very much; Women and illiterate Persons have in some measure contributed to it, by the Discovery of some useful Cures. The Field of Nature is large, and much of it wants still to be cultivated by an ingenious and discreet Application; and the Curious, by their Observations, might daily make further Advances in the History of Nature.

Self-preservation is natural to every living Creature: and thus we see the several Animals of the Sea and the land so careful of themselves, as to observe nicely what is agreeable, and what is hurtful to them; and accordingly they chuse the one, and reject the other.

The Husbandman and the Fisher could expect but little Success without Observation in their several Employments; and it is by Observation that the Physician commonly judges of the Condition of his Patient. A Man of Observation proves often a Physician to himself;

for it was by this that our Ancestors preserv'd their Health till a good old Age, and that Mankind laid up that Stock of natural Knowledg[e], of which they are now possess'd. [3]

Here, Martin draws together the Hippocratic stress on examination of the patient, the adoption of those recommendations by the Gaelic medical school and the inclination to Hippocratic medicine of his mentor Sibbald, and anticipates the medical teaching of the Scottish Enlightenment with its emphasis on clinical medicine – that is, drawing conclusions from observations of individual patients rather than relying on the learning of the lecture hall.

He ends his introduction to the remedies:

> The Wise Solomon did not think it beneath him to write of the meanest Plant, as well as of the tallest Cedar. Hippocrates was at Pains and Charge to travel foreign Countries, with a design to learn the Virtues of Plants, Roots, etc. I have in my little Travels endeavour'd, among other things, in some measure to imitate so great a Pattern: and if I have been so happy as to oblige the Republick of Learning with anything that is useful, I have my Design. I hold it enough for me to furnish my Observations, without accounting for the Reason and Way that those Simples produce them; this I leave to the Learned in that Faculty; and if they would oblige the World with such Theorems from these and the like Experiments, as might serve for Rules upon Occasions of this nature, it would be of great advantage to the Publick. [4]

The simplicity of the remedies employed by the Gaels (and those of the Orcadians and Shetlanders whose customs were also examined) and the general good health of the people in comparison with the diseases prevalent in towns, would not have been lost on Martin's contemporaries. Although the factors of overcrowding, bad housing, poor working conditions, and the lack of proper sewerage systems and safe water supplies underlay the urban health problems, acute illnesses were often exacerbated rather than alleviated by the elaborate concoctions prescribed by physicians and apothecaries. So much so, that the poor who could not afford professional treatment were in some ways better off than the wealthy who succumbed to the fashion for exotic prescriptions.

Martin, however, brought more to the attention of the city doctors than a delightful litany of simple plants and a healthy way of life and diet. He was to record for the first time a then incredible medical theory on susceptibility to disease discovered by the natives of the most remote of all the islands, lonely St Kilda. At first, Martin humbly acknowledges, he was sceptical of the islanders' claims about a condition they called the 'boat cough'. This, the people explained, always coincided with the visit of strangers. The cough was most troublesome at night, when a great deal of phlegm was discharged, and the illness continued for between ten and fourteen days. Once the sovereign remedy was the *gioban* (or *gioban-Iortach*), the fat of fowls stuffed into the stomach of a solan goose and cooked in an infusion of oatmeal. However, they told Martin that this was 'not so effectual now as at the Beginning', a fact they ascribed to its overfrequent use.

In his *A Voyage to St Kilda*, the record of a journey he made in 1697, Martin writes:

> I told them plainly, that I thought all this Notion of Infection but a meer Fancy, and that, at least, it could not always hold; at which they seemed offended, that never any, before the Minister and myself was heard to doubt the Truth of it.[5]

At this the astute St Kildans patiently expanded on their concepts of immunity and their vulnerability to illnesses borne by strangers:

> . . . which is plainly demonstrated upon the landing of every Boat; adding further, that every Design was always for some End, but here there was no room for any, where nothing could be proposed; but for Confirmation of the whole, they appealed to the Case of Infants at the Breast, who were likewise very subject to this Cough, but could not be capable of affecting it, and therefore in their Opinion, they were infected by such as lodged in their Houses. There were scarce

Young or Old in the Isle whom I did not examine particularly upon this Head, and all agreed in the Confirmation of it. They add farther, that when any sovereign Goods are brought thither, then the Cough is of longer Duration than otherwise. They remark, that if the Fever has been among those of the [Macleod of Harris's] Steward's Retinue, though before their Arrival there, some of the Inhabitants are infected with it. If any of the Inhabitants of St Kilda chance to live, though but a short Space, in the Isles of Harries, Skey, or any of the adjacent Isles, they become meagre, and contract such a Cough, that the Giben [*gioban*] must be had, or else they must return to their Native Soil. This Giben is more sovereign for removing of Coughs [as] used by many other Islanders than those of St Kilda. They love to have it frequently in their Meat as well as Drink, by which too frequent Use of it, it is apt to lose its Virtue; it was remarkable, that after this infected Cough was over, we Strangers, and the Inhabitants of St Kilda, making up the Number of about two hundred and fifty, though we had frequently assembled upon the Occasion of Divine Service, yet neither Young nor Old among us all did so much as cough more.[6]

This is as good as an admission, by the end of his stay in the island, that there must be more to the theories behind the 'boat cough' and the reason for the decreasing value of its once 'sovereign remedy' than the 'meer Fancy' of a faraway people.

In addition to this, though possibly unknown to Martin who does not mention it, the Gaels of old had an interesting concept of an inflammation or fever being caused by *grige* (sometimes called *gride*). These are mentioned in various charms and denote, as Dr J.J. Galbraith writes in the *Transactions of the Gaelic Society of Inverness* in 1944, 'a mite, a tiny insect or animalcule, in short a microbe in the original sense'.

In a note on the 'Charm of the Styes' in the *Carmina Gadelica*, Alexander Carmichael wrote:

> It was interesting and instructive to listen to these unlettered old men and women describing 'mar bha mhàthair-ghuir ghrige toir a nìos

a droch àil, ag adhbharachadh buirb agus coirb ann am fuil agus ann am feòil dhaoine' – 'how the hatching mother of the "grig" brought up her bad brood, causing gall and venom in the blood and flesh of people'. Cia mar bha mhàthair-ghuir ghrige faighinn agus a' fàs ann am fuil agus ann am fuil agus ann am feòil neach cha robh e farasda thuigsinn na farasd innseadh; ach aon rud, – far an robh droch thaidhe agus droch ghleidheadh bha ghrige-ghuir an sin, agus i a' ruith bho neach gu neach agus bho theach gu teach mar chleachd an droch sgeula.' – 'How the hatching-mother of the "grig" got into the blood and flesh of a person and grew there it was not easy to understand nor easy to explain; but one thing – where there were ill care and ill keeping the hatching-grig was there, running from person to person and from house to house like the wont of the ill tale (as ill tidings are wont to do).'[7]

The *grig* is not to be confused with the ancient and more widespread idea of a hypothetical 'worm' causing such problems as toothache. Without benefit of the microscope, people had arrived at the concept of *unseen* organisms which not only 'hatched' and proliferated in the body of the afflicted person but could be passed on to the detriment of others.

Science may well have the edge on folk wisdom when it comes to defining microbes and manufacturing antibiotics, but the old Highland notion of the *grig* says everything about how the unfriendly microbes make the victim *feel*. Dr Galbraith remarks in his paper on 'Medicine among the Gaelic Celts': 'This [*grig*] seems not a bad popular exposition of microbic infection and blood poisoning. I have no doubt that there are genuine specimens of the *Eolas* or knowledge of the medieval school of Hebridean physicians [which] anticipate in a vague fashion many modern theories.'

The following description of her method that a healer of *grigean* gave to Carmichael ends with her defending the practice against taunts of witchcraft received when she was living in non-Gaelic Moray. It may help to demonstrate the difference between Highland and Lowland attitudes and why, as will be further explored in the next chapter, unofficial healers were persecuted in the south and north-east but more readily accepted within the Gaelic culture.

Catherine Maclean, a crofter from Naast, near Gairloch, in Wester Ross, begins her narrative with a legend:

> Jesus and His Mother were travelling, and in passing by they went into a house to rest. Who was dwelling in the cottage but a poor widow and three orphans without pith or power. And the poor widow was suffering hard pain from swelling in the breast, and the breast itself was near bursting with swelling.
>
> Jesus asked His Mother to destroy the microbe ['*grig*'] in the pap, and to give peace to the breast and health to the woman. But His Mother said to Christ, 'Do Thou, O Son, destroy the microbe in the pap. It is Thou Thyself, O Son of tears and of sufferings, Who hast received from the Father in heaven power to perform healing on earth.'
>
> There are many things that are crossed (forbidden) and not becoming to do, and it is forbidden to a man to place his hand on a woman's breast. But Christ gave us an example in this matter, as He gave us in many another. Christ blew the warm breath of His mouth on the tortured breast, and He stretched His gentle hand thither over the pap, and he said this verse:

> Extinction to thy microbe,
> Extinction to thy swelling,
> Peace be to thy breast,
> The peace of the King of power.
> Whiteness be to thy skin,
> Subsiding to thy swelling,
> Wholeness to thy breast,
> Fullness to thy pap.
> In the holy presence of the Father,
> In the holy presence of the Son,
> In the holy presence of the Spirit,
> The holy presence of compassion.

No sooner had the Physician of virtues and of blessings uttered these words of power and of virtue than the microbe died, the swelling subsided, and the woman was whole.

Many a great and good thing Christ did on earth, and especially to poor women who were suffering pain and tribulation and shame, in silence of head and in soreness of heart. Many a one that!

I was living in Moray, and I healed the breast-swelling of ten or twelve women while I was there. The people used to mock me, saying that I had witchcraft. But I had no witchcraft, nor anything in creation except the power that God gave me, the God of life and of the worlds, to Whom I prayed to increase my love, to confirm my earnestness, to bless my words and to strengthen my hands. And God did that; the glory be to Him and not to me![8]

Martin Martin, perhaps distancing himself from 'superstition', reported no incantations in his published works. The south knew only the demonology, or supposed demonology, into which many old charms had deteriorated. In comparison, the acceptable Christianised spirituality into which early Highland healers had translated their ancient runes may have been closer to the originals or an improvement on them. The Gaelic versions allowed humility, like that of Catherine Maclean, on the part of the healer, where the verses (many of similar origin) quoted in the Lowland and English witchcraft trials, were often taken as an indication of a desire to control and a show of power. This did not go down well with the authorities.

Perhaps if Martin had collected some of the words along with the simples, that human sense of bonding between healer and patient might also have lent a little influence to the clinical medicine of the Enlightenment.

6

FOLK HEALERS

Unlike other parts of Scotland, the Gaelic-speaking areas remained largely free of the witchcraft persecutions of the sixteenth and seventeenth centuries. Throughout the period there were eighty-nine indictments in the then more populous Highlands and western islands, most of them taking place in the isle of Bute, the eastern seaboards of Ross and Sutherland and in the northern but largely non-Gaelic county of Caithness.[1]

What this meant in terms of traditional healing was a freedom to carry on the old knowledge in a way unparalleled in the rest of the British Isles or much of mainland Europe, where the mania for hunting out 'devilish practices' swept country after country, Protestant and Catholic alike. There certainly were some malevolent or corrupt people who used 'secret' traditions – or late medieval fantasies vaunted as age-old beliefs – to further their own ends, but the complex, and sometimes simply vindictive, motives behind the 'witch'-hunts on the whole seem to have been to thwart those elements in society representing peasant and feminine knowledge which were perceived as a threat to orthodoxy.

Even where Scots-language charms contained Christian references, the Lowland authorities frowned upon them. When Marion (or Margaret) Fisher of Wardie appeared before the kirk session of St Cuthbert's in Edinburgh in 1643 for being a charmer of spells, no witness appeared to accuse her and her judges fell back on the lesser sentence of appointing her to sit in sackcloth in the middle of the church and, before a full congregation, 'to confesse hir charming; and lykeways, *suo consensu*, it is enacted, that if ever schoe be fund to wse any such lyk in tym cuming, to suffer death as ane reall witche'.

One of Marion Fisher's suspect incantations was listed in the session register as:

> Our Lord to hunting red,
> His sooll soot sled;
> Doun he lighted,
> His sool sot righted;
> Blod to blod,
> Shenew to shenew.
> To the other sent in God's name.
> In the name of the Father, Son, and Holy Ghost.[2]

It has many similarities with the bonesetting charm quoted in Chapter 13, the use of which appears to have been perfectly acceptable in Gaelic society.

Childbirth was attended by a host of rituals which, had they continued to be practised with such enthusiasm elsewhere in the British Isles, might have more than doubled the accusations of witchcraft and such fates as befell poor Agnes Sampson, the 'wise wife' of Keith.

She was tried by the High Court in 1590, convicted of curing by 'her develisch prayers', and in the following year burned at the stake for attempting to alleviate the pains of labour. Yet Sampson was described in the *Memoirs* of Sir James Melville (1535–1617) as 'a woman not of the low or ignorant sort of witches, but matron-like, grave and settled in her answers, which were all to some purpose'. The two of her 'develisch prayers' are highly Christian in their tone and, again, not unlike the Gaelic charms in their approach.[3] In another context, such words might have been passed without comment from the Holy Willies who sat in judgement.

Folk knowledge of healing, legend and customs was in a sense the underground, wide-reaching university of the poor and dispossessed. The world-wide interconnection of folklore practices and the underlying themes of its legends do indeed make all people kin. Local variations enhance a sense of regional or national identity. It was a danger that authoritarian institutions recognised with, ironically, perhaps the same intuition that informed the traditions themselves.

Among the Gaels such knowledge was to survive not as the province of the outcast but within the natural context of a pre-industrial society. Although in later times some of the clergy would mutter in despair of heathen ways, others were to be interested collectors of the old customs, recognising them as a genuine repository of the people's ancient history.[4]

Nevertheless, there *was* a dark and sinister side which is best dealt with before looking at the far wider Highland scene of benign healing. The case of Hector Monro, seventeenth Baron of Foulis, who was brought to trial in Easter Ross in July 1590, is not only an extreme and fortunately rare – in Scottish annals, at least – example of what might truly be called black magic but serves to show that 'justice' could favour the highborn and well-to-do, however bizarre or revolting the crime. Munro and several others, including his stepmother, were charged with sorcery, incantation, witchcraft, and slaughter.

When Hector fell sick in 1588 he sent for a notorious witch, Marion Macingaruch, who administered three draughts of water in which three stones had been infused. When this did not work she told Munro there would be no remedy unless the principal man of his blood should suffer death for him. His half-brother, George, was the chosen victim. After a grotesque catalogue of events which included a symbolic burial of Hector, a dialogue with his 'maister the devill', libations of milk, honey and the blood of sacrificed animals in the name of pagan deities, George Munro was 'seized with a mortal distemper' in April 1590 and died two months later.

Hector and Lady Foulis were the only two accused to be acquitted; several of the others were executed; the fate of yet others – including Marion Macingaruch, though convicted, remains unknown.[5] Of the whole nasty business, even the dirt-digging John Graham Dalyell remarks in his *The Darker Superstitions of Scotland*: 'No ceremony alike remarkable is recorded in Scottish history; nor is it obvious from what combination of sources, either in theory or practice it was derived.'[6]

There seems little doubt, however, that the ritual sacrifice of bulls still being carried out in Wester Ross in the latter half of the seventeenth century derived from the druidic sacrifices of bulls described by Pliny and the early Gaelic chroniclers.

Among 'abominable and heathinishe practizes' minuted by a presbytery meeting at Applecross in 1656, was information that a number of men from Achnashellach had sacrificed a bull, walked sunwise about ruined chapels, and predicted future events by a hollowed round stone into which 'they tryed the entreing of thair head' on 25 August, St Maelrubha's feast day. In 1678 the presbytery of Dingwall recorded that Hector Mackenzie, with two sons and a grandson, had sacrificed a bull 'in ane heathenish manner on Eilean Ma-Ruibhe (Innis Maree) for this sake of his wife Cirstane's health'. Since the minutes describe this woman as '*formerlie* sick and valetudinairie,' the ritual might just have had some psychological effect.[7]

The island in Loch Maree was an ancient and possibly even pre-Christian healing sanctuary which has many traditions attached to it (see Chapter 10). In the 1678 incident, it was claimed in the presbytery minutes, the men had offered their sacrifice not to the Christian saint of the area, Maelrubha, but on the site of an ancient temple in honour of a being whom some called 'St Mourie' and others 'ane god Mourie'. Bull symbolism was frequently associated with the healing and oracular sanctuaries of the ancient Celts.

By the end of the seventeenth century, the old Gaelic social order was well into decline and the increasingly southern-leaning aspirations of the chiefs and their families had as little room for the old learning as their descendants were to have for the many ordinary people who were cleared from their homes a century and more later.

The Macleods of Harris, whose seat was – and still is – at Dunvegan Castle in Skye, had, along with the Macdonalds, been leading patrons of the old learned orders, but already by the 1660s the domestic accounts show payments made to Lowland doctors. One of the most interesting is a fee of £13 14s Scots (£1 2s 10d sterling) paid to a Dr Brisbane for a consultation.[8]

In the 1660s, the chief who consulted this doctor (who may have been the Glasgow physician, Dr Matthew Brisbane, who gave evidence at the Renfrew witch trial of 1697 where he affirmed his views that witchcraft and 'compacts with the devil' could cause illnesses) was the seventeenth chief, Ruairidh Mear, Roderick the Witty, variously described by his contemporaries as a 'prodigal vitious spendthrift' (the opinion of a Fraser) and 'a man of uncommon liveliness and wit' (a fellow Macleod's assessment), and in reality perhaps all of these things. A chemist's bill for 1661 tells of a Dunvegan household much plagued by constipation, insomnia, headaches and depression – enough to make any man a spendthrift or, indeed, the prodigality may itself have brought on the foregoing problems.

He kept a good table, ordering, as well as the venison, beef and salmon of his own country, spices by the pound, oranges and lemons by the dozen and prunes, understandably, by the stone. Orders for syrup of white poppies and 'ane lairg somniferaus emulsion' (for sleeping), diuretics (for the kidneys), and aperitifs, cordials and purges galore tell of a household that relished its wine and spiced meat. Much of Ruairidh's time was spent living it up in the south, especially in Edinburgh, where he greatly increased the debt on the estate. By 1664 he had burnt himself out and was dead at the age of twenty-eight with no direct heir – his only son, Norman, having predeceased him. Fortunately for the Macleods he was succeeded by his brother, Iain Breac, who, while of equally poor constitution, was described as a 'most hopeful, excellent and wise youth'.

In the 1690s there was a man living at Husabost in Skye, not far from the Macleod seat at Dunvegan Castle, who did indeed draw suspicions of witchcraft upon himself, perhaps indirectly through those new southern influences on the local chiefs, perhaps through the growing influence of the church.

Neil Beaton was described by Martin Martin as an 'illiterate Empirick', but in all likelihood Neil was well-learned in the context of a powerful oral tradition in which the faculty of memory was cultivated in a manner lost to us today.

Since Neil appears to have inherited the practical tradition of the official medieval doctors and was unencumbered by the medical literature of the time, it is worth quoting Martin's observation of him in full for the light it sheds on unofficial healing methods:

[Neil Beaton] of late is so well known in the Iles and Continent, for his great success in curing several dangerous Distempers, tho he never appeared in the quality of a *Physician* until he arrived at the Age of Forty Years, and then also without the advantage of Education. He pretends to judg of the various qualities of Plants, and Roots, by their different Tastes; he has likewise a nice Observation of the Colours of their Flowers, from which he learns their astringent and loosening qualities: he extracts the Juice of Plants and Roots, after a Chymical way, peculiar to himself, and with little or no charge.

He considers his Patients Constitution before any Medicine is administered to them; and he has form'd such a System for curing Diseases, as serves for a Rule to him upon all Occasions of this nature.

He treats *Riverius's Lilium Medicinae*, and some other Practical Pieces that he has heard of, with Contempt; since in several Instances it appears that their Method of Curing has fail'd, where his had good Success.

Some of the Diseases cured by him are as follows: Running Sores in Legs and Arms, grievous Head-aches; he had the boldness to cut a piece out of a Woman's skull broader than half a Crown, and by this restor'd her to perfect Health. A Gentlewoman of my Acquaintance having contracted a dangerous Pain in her Belly, some days after her

Delivery of a Child, and several Medicines being us'd, she was thought past recovery, if she continued in that Condition a few hours longer; at last this Doctor happen'd to come there, and being imploy'd, apply'd a Simple Plant to the part affected, and restored the Patient in a quarter of an hour after the Application.

One of his Patients told me that he sent him a Cap interlined with some Seeds, &c. to wear for the Cough, which it remov'd in a little time; and it had the like effect upon his Brother.

The Success attending this Man's Cures was so extraordinary, that several People thought his Performances to have proceeded rather from a Compact with the Devil, than from the Virtue of Simples. To obviate this, Mr *Beaton* pretends [i.e. claims] to have had some Education from his Father, tho he died when he himself was but a Boy. I have discours'd him seriously at different times, and am fully satisfied, that he uses no unlawful means for obtaining his end.

His Discourse of the several Constitutions, the Qualities of Plants, &c. was more solid than could be expected from one of his Education. Several sick People from remote Iles came to him; and some from the Shire of *Ross*, at 70 miles distance, sent for his Advice: I left him very successful, but can give no further Account of him since that time.[9]

Martin took pains to defend Beaton's reputation at some length, showing concern to present him as an 'honest broker'. The portrait provides sufficient evidence for a genuine, knowledgeable healer practising on the borderline between the already outdated orthodox medicine of the Middle Ages and the folk practice that largely filled the gap until the establishment of a proper medical system in the Highlands which was not to be fully implemented until the early twentieth century.

As elsewhere, there had always been unofficial healers and doubtless they had their place even during the years when the formally educated physicians held sway, but they truly came into their own in the Highlands during the late seventeenth century and throughout the eighteenth, with diminishing influence into the beginning of the twentieth. Largely unhampered by taunts of witchcraft (provided they kept in with their neighbours), firmly ensconced in a tradition-minded society, and geographically remote from the influences of city ways, they were to keep alive a form of medicine which in other parts of Europe was either to become inextricably confused with 'dark doings' – and a prey to corruption by those with a fancy for the occult – or disappear from all but the most isolated peasant communities.

The word 'folk' sits awkwardly in the context of Gaelic society, the very term implying a dichotomy in cultural interests between the 'educated', the 'cultured' and the genteel, and the ways of the common people. In Highland society, even for some time after the anglicisation processes of the seventeenth century, the culture was held in common between the people, their chiefs and the tacksmen.

The local healers, of diverse types and backgrounds, interweave the practical with the mythological and it is in their work that the sense of historical and multi-cultural 'healing threads' most truly come into play, particularly in the incantations and rituals used.

> Fhir tha marcachd an eich bhric,
> Ciod as leigheas air an t-sruth-chasd?
> (Rider of the piebald horse,
> What is a cure for whooping cough?)[10]

was a question asked of strangers on horseback in the belief that they had the power of recommending the correct remedy. It is possible to see in this practice an echo of the ancient cult of a Celtic Apollo, a healer and solar god, frequently depicted on horseback. But this deity had, in a sense, a medieval Scottish counterpart in James IV, during whose reign much of Scotland, including the peasantry, prospered. He made frequent and extensive horseback tours throughout the country, Highland and Lowland alike, and his passion for medicine also brought him respect for his skills in surgery and dentistry. He was also noted for his almsgiving to the poor. As such he was a folk hero, reinforcing the mythology of the rider as healer. Is it just coincidence that the Greek father of medicine, Hippocrates, whose school of medical writing was often quoted by the clan physicians, had a name which means 'he who holds the horse'?

However, the quacks and charlatans who travelled by horse to ply their dubious trade in later centuries must have brought a great deal of disillusion along with their pink pills and green potions.

While royalty and the otherwise high and mighty were resorted to for the healing touch in the Highlands as elsewhere in Europe, there were other people who were believed to have such power by virtue of who they were rather than what they knew.

Names could be important. A condition known as *glacach*, indicated by a tightness and fullness in the chest, was treated by certain families of Macdonalds who stroked the chest and murmured incantations. If any fee were offered or accepted, the cure was said to be ineffectual. It was also said that putting a child sick with whooping-cough to nurse in a family in which the husband and wife were of the same name before marriage – a not uncommon occurrence in Gaeldom – would effect a cure.

The clergy were credited with the power of curing epilepsy and bishops in particular were supposed to cure insanity as well, especially that variety in which the victim's heart was believed to be 'out of place'. A Beauly doctor recounted that in his area the power was exclusively vested in Roman Catholic priests. Although he was writing in the late nineteenth century he was, like so many who collected the old cures of the period, also recalling the last vestiges of much more widespread practices from earlier times:

> I have heard various cases cited. One remains particularly distinct in my memory. The patient was an elderly woman, the mother of Jenny the dressmaker, and during a professional visit of the daughter to our house, I surreptitiously overheard the tale. The mother had suffered for some time from the almost unnamable malady [epilepsy], and as a result of considerable persuasion she was induced to visit the priest at Beauly, whose healing powers were well known.

He received her kindly, and with solemn ceremony invested her with a cord covered with beads, which she was to wear round her neck both night and day, nor for any reason whatever remove it till the hour of her death. She returned, and for a considerable time all went well. But one day – whether for the purpose of extraordinary ablution, or from failing faith, or by the instigation of the devil, did not exactly appear, but all were suggested to my mind by the narrative – one day she temporarily removed the sacred necklet, and it was by no means long thereafter that a fit of fearful violence came on, in which the patient was terrible to behold, and this seizure either terminated in, or was speedily followed by, death.[11]

The healing power of the seventh son of a seventh son is well attested not only in Celtic folklore but even in lingering present-day belief, with the well-known Irish healer, Finbarr Nolan, having launched his vocation on the strength of being the seventh son of a seventh son. The potency of such a belief has been such that only the modern custom of smaller families will soon mean that it becomes part of the history rather than the practice of folklore. Seventh daughters also carried on the tradition in some parts of Ireland and Scotland. In Caithness and Sutherland it was claimed a seventh son could cure the King's Evil (scrofula) in a woman, and a seventh daughter could do the same for a man, while the seventh son of a seventh son might cure all kinds of diseases. In her *Folksongs and Folklore of South Uist*, Margaret Fay Shaw writes that the seventh child of a line of either boys or girls inherited the power to cure scrofula and she instances a young Uist girl and a Glasgow boy of a Highland family who went to Barra for the cure in 1932.

The cure of scrofulous disorders – which in former times included every form of chronic discharging sore as well as glandular problems – by the power of incantations, the touch of kings, or the seventh sons of seventh sons was widely believed. The ritual varied according to time and place, but the records of the Caledonian Medical Society give a late nineteenth century example personally known to one of its own members, a doctor in Inverness.

The patient was a man of about sixty who suffered from a keloid (an outgrowth of fibrous tissue) on his neck. Having been subjected to most of the orthodox modes of treatment without much benefit, he took the advice of some friends and repaired to a seventh son of a seventh son who lived some ten miles from Inverness. This 'rustic Aesculapius', as the doctor calls him, informed the patient that the cure would occupy three days, and on the first day the treatment consisted in spitting saliva on the affected part and thoroughly rubbing it into the flesh. This was repeated on the second and third days. Before he left, the man was given three bottles filled with a clear, odourless fluid, which, it was directed, were to be used for cleansing the sores thrice daily, and when one third empty to be filled with water. This was to be continued till three bottles of each had been used, when the cure would be complete. The man told the doctor that he had carried out these instructions most carefully, with the result, after three months, that the condition of his neck was the same as before.

Even the manner in which people were born, never mind their or their father or mother's place in the family pecking order, could be significant. Breech or footling births presaged a baby who would grow up with the power of curing epilepsy or injuries to the back or spine and, in some areas, rheumatism. To be born with the caul attached also gave healing powers and very often the caul was preserved throughout the person's lifetime as an especially lucky amulet. A child born after the death of its father was also said to be endowed with the power to heal.

Some people were said to be gifted with easing inflammations of the eye by rubbing the affected organ with a stone on which he or she had spat and sprinkled soot. Others were supposed to be able to arrest any flux or haemorrhage by repeating certain words and administering a bowl of the patient's own blood, boiled, dried and powdered, a practice which was once, apparently, quite popular.

Folk medicine was where women came into their own. Their responsibility for diagnosis and the carrying out of treatment at a time when professionals were few and far between, showed a high measure of understanding and intelligence, and only as a last resort would the doctor – if one were available – be called.

As well as astute mothers, wives and aunts, a kind of unique specialist had evolved among the Highland womenfolk, the *cailleach chearc* or henwife, who was much resorted to for midwifery, charms against toothache and the numerous incantations believed to dispel every kind of sickness and difficulty.

A prominent figure in many old Gaelic stories, the henwife rarely drew even flippant accusations of witchcraft, however arcane-seeming her knowledge, and she was often taken under the wing of the chief or the laird for protection.

Mrs Katherine Whyte Grant, a Highland-born translator and author of plays for children, told the Caledonian Medical Society in 1904:

> Those who have listened to Gaelic tales, told and re-told, cannot fail to have been puzzled by the important place assigned to her. She is resorted to for love potions, for charms, for advice on setting out upon an expedition – in short, she it is who guides almost all affairs to a happy issue, or at least brings about the desires of those who consult her, working such mischief in the families of those who hinder the good fortune of her clients.

The general impression one has of the henwife is of a neat and clean, middle-aged to elderly woman quietly and firmly dispensing care, advice, medicine and comfort.

At the other end of the scale were the so-called 'witches'.[12] Very often they were women, though there were men among them, who had fallen on bad times and used what knowledge they had in order to survive. If they could benefit by emphasising their eccentricities, then some did so. The Caithness 'witch' of Ballachly, the 'Fitheach' mentioned in Chapter 2, may have been typical. No one knew where she was from, or even what her real name was. In her old age she just wandered into her hovel near Rangag and made her livelihood partly by begging from house to house, and partly by using her peculiar knowledge.

It is likely that such women were the ones resorted to by those, especially unmarried girls, seeking an abortion. Although it was not uncommon for a course of purgatives to be taken every autumn and spring in order to adapt the body to the change of season, several of the herbal 'remedies' allegedly taken by women for that purpose would have been excessively violent.

James Robertson, who toured the West Highlands and some of the islands in 1768, noted:

> The women are frequently troubled with a suppression of the menses, to remedy which they use an infusion of the Thalictrum minus and the Linum catharticum. The Lycopodium selago is said to be such a strong purge that it will bring on an abortion.[13]

In fact, all three plants mentioned have been used at some time as abortifacients. Unlike many contemporary travellers in the Highlands, Robertson delved deep into basic details and seems to have had a deft way of eliciting confidences regarding women's problems. He also mentions the epidemics of 'sibbens' (syphilis) which, although they had abated by the time of his travels, particularly afflicted the Highlands in the first half of the eighteenth century, having been brought in by miners in the 1730s and soldiers in the 1740s.

Bone-setters were specialists among the unofficial healers and even where there was access to professional care, there was a widespread belief that the treatment of bone and joint injuries lay outside the province of the regular medical practitioner, and that the bone-setter was the only safe person to be entrusted with the cure. Physicians, such as Dr J. R. Logan writing in the *Caledonian Medical Journal* in 1896, were sceptical:

I have known several persons who were treated by a famous exponent of that art in our neighbourhood, and in two cases I happen to know fairly definitely the nature of the injury, the treatment and the result. In one there was fracture of the olecranon; in the other the neck of the femur was broken. In both cases there was first a very vigorous *taxis* used, and this was followed by the continuous application of tow and white of egg. The results were, of course, highly unsatisfactory.[14]

Patients who resorted to bonesetters, however, seemed satisfied enough, and not all physicians were as dubious as Logan. Dr Donald Masson, writing in the *Transactions of the Gaelic Society of Inverness*, told from personal experience how the bone-setters' special skill in treating dislocations involved constant watching for indications of pain and in locking the knee or elbow joint straight in order to provide extra thrust at the critical moment.[15] Among the last practitioners on the mainland were Simon MacBean or MacBain, of Milton of Balnagowan near Ardersier, and Donald Munro, of Knockancuirn near Evanton, and an excellent account of them is given in Frank Maclennan's *Ferindonald Papers*, published by Ross & Cromarty Heritage Society.

Where men tended to specialise in fractures, each area had its women who were skilled in manipulation and massage. Like the men, they asked no fee but the butter they used as a lubricant. Manipulation was often used in the Highlands as a way of treating tuberculosis, a part of the diagnosis of which was the behaviour of the sputum when expectorated on to a level surface. If it fell flat it was regarded as a positive sign of tuberculosis, while if it broke and scattered the disease was not consumption.

The lungs were forcibly expanded by drawing the lower ribs outwards with the hands oiled with fresh butter, the operator standing behind the patient, who was seated in a chair before a fire. In Stratherrick a similar mode of treatment was used for rickets but in addition the body was raised by drawing the clavicle and head upwards. During treatment the patient was advised to drink as much milk, especially that of the goat, donkey or mare as possible. In lumbago and other back pains the patient lay flat on the floor, and the barefoot attendant massaged the spine by taking short steps backwards and forwards on his back.

The risks attendant on a woman in labour led to a multiplicity of protective customs. At one time the mother took out double insurance with pagan and Christian spirits by having a piece of cold iron with her in the bed, and a Bible below her pillow. The midwife would see if every lock in the house was open in case some charm (from an ill-wisher) was hidden in the keyhole. Before the child was washed, the midwife would take the straw from under the mother and, having made a rope of part of it, divided it into three parts. It was then thrown on the fire to be consumed along with any evil that might afterwards be wished against the child. In winter the infant was taken outside and a mark was made in the snow with its bare foot as a further safeguard against troubles. A burning peat might be carried round the bed sunwise seven times. If this were impracticable owing to restricted space or the position of the bed, then it was deemed sufficient to encircle the outside of the house.

Charms and rituals to prevent fairies stealing or exchanging babies for one of their own were many and various, but the following story, witnessed by a medical man towards the end of the nineteenth century and recounted to the Caledonian Medical Society by Katherine Whyte Grant, has similarities with a ritual mentioned by Thomas Pennant over a hundred years earlier and may, in origin, have been extremely ancient:

> Hugh's son and heir was born about eight of a winter evening. Hugh was from home, but the old seer was hovering about the house door. He was hale, erect, and white-haired, a fine old figure for a man of nearly ninety. The seer's daughter, Sheila, was nurse, and Evir, the stately grand-parent, was superintending the household. Doctor R. was in attendance. After the mother was made comfortable with a glass of whisky and a piece of oatcake, the seer was called into the kitchen; also Hector, the foxhunter, and Norman. Evir laid the babe in the

arms of the seer. 'We must have the child baptised after the ancient manner,' said they. By her father's instructions, Sheila brought a tub of water and set it on the hearth in their midst. The seer poured three glasses of whisky and three of wine into the water; he then added three spoonfuls of salt. Three short swords were laid in the tub, then all formed a circle around the hearth. The seer placed the child in Hector's arms, as being next of kin. Hector gave him to Norman, and Norman returned him to Evir, who, along with Sheila, stood godmother to the boy. Evir washed the babe in the bath prepared by the seer, and said, as she did so, 'I name thee M., in the presence of these thy godfathers and thy godmothers, and in the presence of the invisible, all-seeing Father. I pray to him to protect thee from the evil desires of thine enemies, and the evil desires of the enemies of thy forefathers.' Then Evir went to the room and laid the child by his mother.

'What are we to do for milk?' asked the doctor. Evir went to the door and gave a peculiar call. Her white doe, with its fawn, came bounding up to her. She milked the doe, and brought her milking to the doctor. 'Excellent,' he exclaimed, 'there could be nothing better.' A little was poured into a cup, a few drops of whisky added, and a little honey, and the whole thoroughly mixed, and the babe was fed with it by Evir. Then she and Sheila send a round of mountain dew and oatcake to each family in the clachan, that they might drink to the health of Hugh's heir.

One peculiarity may be mentioned here. The name given by Evir was not the name by which the boy was known as he grew up, though the seer and she continued so to designate him.[16]

The Celtic smith-god Gobniu had mystical associations with healing and until well into the nineteenth century the blacksmith was called upon to help in such matters as the drawing of teeth and attending on ritual cures. In the days when the clan physicians held sway over medicine, the smiths held a high status as clan armourers and often figured in tales of heroism and romance. As with the physicians they were given free land and other privileges. In the breakdown of the old system their work, though increasingly agricultural rather than military, continued to be of such necessity and value that they retained their standing in the community.

Many families of smiths were hereditary, and not just in Gaeldom – a fact which has, in various linguistic forms, given rise to arguably the most familiar surname in Europe. They had staying-power and, no doubt due to their steady incomes, were able to nourish large and sturdy families. In the residual Celtic areas of Ireland, Wales and the Scottish Highlands they also retained their traditional semi-magical significance longer than elsewhere. Down the ages certain families of smiths perfected a treatment for depression which not only required considerable skill and accuracy but seems to have anticipated later electric-shock remedies for psychiatric cases.

At the end of the seventeenth century Martin Martin recorded the method of a smith in the Skye parish of Kilmartin who was reputed as 'a Doctor for curing Faintness of the Spirits'. He was the thirteenth generation of his family to practise both the trade and this particular cure:

> The Patient being laid on the Anvil with his Face uppermost, the Smith takes a big Hammer in both his Hands, and making his Face all Grimace, he approaches his Patient; and as if he design'd to hit him with his full Strength on the Forehead, he ends in a Feint, else he would be sure to cure the Patient of all Diseases: but the Smith being accustom'd to the Performance, has a Dexterity of managing his Hammer with Discretion; tho at the same time he must do it so as to strike Terror in the Patient: and this they say has always the design'd Effect. [17]

Sometimes harsh, sometimes extravagant, sometimes, from our point of view, simply strange, such rituals must have had some influence if only from the sense of drama created. The seemingly bizarre methods employed for treating epilepsy in particular may have originated in the belief that the drama would somehow activate the brain into another mode. At the very least, the scenarios would have been memorable and their enactment was evidence of the respect given to the power of the mind in the healing process. It is possible that such dramas represented a 'rite of passage' between sickness and health and reinforced the patient's confidence and will to recover.

A cure for epilepsy practised in the Western Isles in 1909 and recorded by George Henderson in his *Norse Influence on Celtic Scotland*, contains in one grand performance many of the individual aspects of epilepsy remedies practised elsewhere.

After two years of receiving professional treatment for his epilepsy in Edinburgh, the patient went to see a healer in Lewis.[18] Blood was taken from the patient's left foot, and given him (the patient) to drink. The healer then cut a piece of nail from each finger and toe of the patient, some hairs from the eyebrows and moustache, and wrapped them in papers.

Three straw ropes of the length of the patient's body were made, and then another three of the length of the patient's out-stretched hands and body. These ropes were put crosswise on the body of the sufferer with their ends folded and knotted. The knots were then cut and the cuttings put in papers, and the whole contents buried in a place where neither sun nor wind nor rain could get at them.

A black cock was to be buried at the spot where the patient had the fit for the first time. The sufferer was also directed to drink out of a *copan-cinn* (skull-pan) taken from an old cemetery on a small island, which he did for some weeks, reporting to Henderson that 'the peculiar taste was fresh in the mouth the next morning as it was on the previous night'.

The patient, a respectable Free Church man, admitted that during this treatment, if he was not better, he was not much worse. He had not heard the words of the incantation, but he saw the lips of the healer, 'this survivor of a long line of medical-men' move as he repeated the charms to himself. 'And with kindly thoughts towards this old-world rite, with simple heart, he once more set out for Edinburgh.'

Henderson commented: 'I felt much moved as the sufferer told me this and in touch with ages almost as distant as when the glorious mountains were brought forth that I then gazed upon, and near by were children's young voices and the sea's mysterious murmur. An old shepherd was present and – inexpressible to myself – my thoughts were at the heart of things.'[19]

Fire was a not uncommon part of remedial dramas. A story was told of a young girl who had sickened for months with a disease that was 'slowly wearing her to her grave'. Local doctors had practically given up her case as hopeless and her parents were desperate. The child was taken to a remote glen where a circle of fire was made and she was carefully passed from hand to hand through the ring of fire to the cadence of an ancient *rann*. From that day, it was said, the girl grew in health and strength and ultimately completely recovered. Often it was babies, ailing or otherwise, who were passed through the circle of fire which might be a ring of burning peats and logs on the ground or a fiery hoop supported in the air.

'Rickets' was a name often applied to a disease which appears to have similarities with the modern eating afflictions of anorexia and bulimia. The symptoms, which were described by a doctor over a hundred years ago as attacking young women and servant girls more than any other class of the community, included 'a weariness of the limbs, and a general languor of mind and body. The bright eye lost its lustre; there was a loathing of food; the heart was undoubtedly affected, and respiratory disturbance was indicated by frequent and deep sighing.'

No herb was known that had any effect on it and its cure baffled even the renowned skills of the 'wise women'. Dr J R Logan, the same man who was dismissive of bone-setters, wrote in the *Caledonian Medical Journal* that there was only one resort:

> The maiden was to be taken to a 'knowing man', who had a secret remedy which would remove her trouble. His mode of procedure I

could never find out exactly, but I understand he did something in the way of massage of the ribs [Logan thinks similar to that resorted to in tuberculosis] . . . I further can certify that one of our domestics visited a practitioner of this kind at the Muir of Ord, and that she returned materially improved and greatly comforted.[20]

A colleague of Logan's, Dr Alastair Macgregor, lent credence to the folk belief that jaundice could be cured by giving the patient a fright by dashing cold water over the naked body or suddenly 'threatening' the patient by holding a red-hot iron close to the spine:

I well remember a patient of mine who had jaundice from a sluggish liver, which did not improve satisfactorily under the ordinary methods of treatment, being set on the high road to recovery by one of his neighbour's children, who had a grudge against him, throwing a lighted cracker into the room in which he was sleeping. The patient got a tremendous fright, vomited profusely, and began mending ever after.[21]

A 'distance-healing' method of healing sore eyes may owe more to a method still practised by some north Highland mothers than to anything mystical. William Don was a fisherman in Latheronwheel, Caithness, whose speciality was the removing of grit or any foreign matter out of people's eyes. It was said he would remove the irritant without touching the eye with hand or instrument, and it was immaterial whether the person was present or not. A local minister, the Revd George Sutherland, wrote in 1937: 'He, no doubt, used mystical formulae, and as a finish off he would take a mouthful of water and spout it out into his hand, and the hurtful matter that had been in the eye would now be in William's hand.' Reports of the man's methods, however, may have been misunderstood. It was common practice in the north for the healer, especially in the case of a mother of a child, to lick the foreign body out with her tongue. This may have been William Don's 'no-hands-on' method.

Fascinating though some of the stranger-seeming methods are, herbal infusions and poultices and the use of other material medicines, as well as sweating cures and the visiting of wells, made up by far the bulk of the old remedies, a wide range of which is given in Part II.

Idiosyncratic rituals are not unique to folk medicine and exist, in more subtle forms, even in modern orthodox medicine. Not for nothing is the operating room of a hospital known as the 'theatre'. The dramas of life and death, sickness and health and mental stress, and all the human emotions these involve, are what medicine is all about. By involving the patient in an artificially created drama, the unofficial healer was probably trying to present the abstract, unknowable force of the disease in concrete terms; and by holding up, as it were, a mirror to reality, allowing the patient to come to grips with something more tangible. Not all psychiatry had its origins in nineteenth-century Vienna.

7

LAIRDS, MINISTERS
AND DOMINIES

In the long years between the dispersal of the clan physicians and the introduction of the Highlands & Islands Medical Scheme in 1919, virtually only the well-off and those who lived in or near towns and larger villages, and the utterly destitute – who were to have basic provision under the Poor Law Amendment Act of 1845 – had any access to professional medical care, and, as the Dewar Report of 1912 was to show, even that could vary greatly in quality.

The travelling peddlers of 'miracle cures' were usually next to useless, although they appear to have provided a certain sadistic entertainment (to onlookers) with their efforts at dentistry. Only the local unofficial healers maintained, according to their own traditions, a sense of dependability and their services were usually free or occasionally paid for in kind, more from gratitude than for the asking.

For about a hundred years from the last decades of the eighteenth century, a fourth type of healing became prominent in the advice and help of lairds, ministers and dominies whose medical knowledge was almost entirely gained from books, many of which were of a decidedly dubious nature. If the calibre of treatment could vary greatly among the qualified practitioners, where they were to be found in rural areas, voluntary arrangements with the local gentry, clergy and dominies could be even more haphazard and very much dependent on the benevolence of relationships as well as the healer's knowledge.

The old *Statistical Accounts* of the 1790s, submitted mainly by ministers, include comments on local health conditions and many of the measures, traditional and currently orthodox, taken for treating illness. If the varying remarks of these men on the character of their parishioners is anything to go by – one parish might be full of God-fearing, near-angelic folk yet the neighbouring minister might deplore the heathen ways of his flock – attitude and application depended very much on the individual.

Yet these were also the years when the great Highland regiments were formed, bodies of men renowned for their stamina and strength under duress and their courage on the battlefield.

The certain cynicism that channelled the Gaels' innate sense of loyalty and determination into the armed services to the benefit of an Empire whose ethos had contributed to the demise of their own society, largely ignored the heritage that had produced those men and the communities who fostered them. The more rousing music of the bagpipe and the swing of the kilt were fine. They encouraged the martial spirit, bonded regimental brotherhood and even began to excite a new sense of Scottishness in those Lowlanders with no Highland connections, whose recent forebears would have spurned the rumoured barbarity of the Gael and what was seen as an impenetrable language.

Ironically, the more intense the promotion of the tartan and its connections with matters military and romantic, the more rapid became the decline of other aspects of the old order such as the clarsach, a more truly Gaelic instrument but one which did not lend itself to martial airs. Formal education, in particular, served to create the chasm. It divorced the Gaels from many of the cultural strengths of their own past, once shared by proud and humble alike, without introducing them to similar standards in the new culture. As Derick Thomson has written:

The introduction of English, first of all to the southerly and eastern communities, introduced Gaels, not to the glories of English literature but to the simpler ephemera of the elementary schoolroom, to the chapbook and to the models of semi-literate taste. All this is reflected in the 'new' Gaelic verse of the nineteenth century, which largely turns its back on its own relatively learned, aristocratic tradition, and grovels contentedly in its novel surroundings.[1]

They are well-aimed words which he qualifies by adding, 'As always, there were survivals from the older order, individuals who made an effort to cling to the tradition.' Such poets may be compared with those pipers who kept alive the *Ceòl Mòr*, the classical music of the bagpipe, when encouragement was being channelled in the direction of regimental marches and the dances newly discovered by the southern gentry. It was in the keeping of that tradition by the few, that the best Gaelic poets of our times have been able to draw a strength and move the literature forward into a vibrant modern idiom.

The survival of medical traditions traces a different path. Throughout the eighteenth century the old ways were subject to a continual process of erosion, but the upheavals of the post-Culloden Highlands from 1746 on were probably not as severe a threat to traditional medicine as they were to other areas of life.

The tacksman or middle-class stratum of Gaelic society still shared a common cultural inheritance with the humblest cottars – with one vital difference. The tacksman class was more likely to be literate in Gaelic as well as English and to act as a buffer not only between aristocrat and cottar, but also between the old ways and the new. Its departure in phases from the 1730s to the 1820s, with a surge of voluntary emigrations in the last decade of the eighteenth century, was to leave a gulf between the poorer peasantry and the landowners that undoubtedly made the enforced clearances of the next century easier to pursue. The vacuum was all the worse for occurring in a society that had, since time immemorial, been constructed on a strictly hierarchical basis. While there had been an admirable equality of discourse and the vitality of a shared culture between all ranks of that society, it was also one in which everyone knew their place. Hereditary orders, like those of the pipers, bards, clerics, genealogists, legal and medical men, needed a strong agricultural base – chiefly linked to cattle – to sustain the economy. Deprived of ancestral social sanction, the practice of the old healing tradition might have disappeared along with many of the other old ways if it had not become an economic necessity.

The highly structured Celtic society of Iron Age Europe which had suited the Highlands so well and for so long was not easily shaken off in the people's attitudes. That vacuum left by the departure of the enterprising, one might call it 'managerial', style of the tacksmen was to some extent filled by the landowners, the church and schoolteachers. As with the tacksmen, the people's proper pride did not rate them any more highly as human beings – and in time they were, justifiably, to rate some landowners considerably lower – but they were looked on, if not necessarily up to, as educated people.

Schools, especially those set up by the Society for the Propagation of Christian Knowledge, attracted teachers to some of the more remote areas, ministers were installed in isolated parishes that may have had little or no formal religious leadership for a century or more, and, together with the bigger farmers and the lairds themselves, such people represented almost the only small core of an elite.

Self-help became not only the fashion but the necessity. (At one time there was only one qualified medical practitioner in the whole of Sutherland, a county of over 2000 square miles.) Where the poorer people still resorted to the fields and hillsides for herbal medicines, the use of the personal medicine chest came into its own in the houses of the new middle class. Sulphur, aloes and senna were among the medicines they kept in stock and there was a firm belief in the benefits of salts, a fact which may speak volumes about purgative attitudes in other areas of life. Nevertheless, where the clergy saw it as their duty to care for bodies as well as souls and teachers helped to sort physical ills as well as improving minds, lairds and their womenfolk – especially the womenfolk – often showed more responsibility than their image allows them.

Although no exact area was given for the following incident related in 1896 by Dr Duncan Macgregor to the Caledonian Medical Society, he was born and brought up in Inverness-shire in the first half of the nineteenth century and it may well have taken place in that county. The doctor averred the story to be 'perfectly true':

> A lady in the Highlands, learning that a man (one of her tenants) was ill, went to see him. The patient looked bad, and his trouble evidently lay in his chest. As no doctor was in attendance, the lady advised the man's wife to poultice, and, in answer to the query as to what best to be applied, recommended carrots. Next day, on calling, the lady was surprised to see the man lying in bed with his chest covered with what looked like pieces of wet paper. On asking for an explanation she was electrified by the man's wife saying, 'Well, your ladyship, I put on as many Catechisms as I could get, but there were not nearly enough, so I made out with the *Pilgrim's Progress*'. It was evident that . . . the woman mistook what was ordered, and not having Catechisms enough at hand, supplemented what she had with the next best 'good book'. And so the *Pilgrim's Progress* was stewed and applied – truly one of the most unique old Highland remedies on record.[2]

The story has not been chosen simply as an anecdotal curiosity but as an entwiner of various contemporary threads. It is taken as quite natural that it should be the lady of the estate, and not a physician, who is advising the tenant. She prescribes a carrot poultice (then highly regarded in rural medicine for cancerous sores), showing an instant knowledge of what might be beneficial. She is caring and makes a follow-up visit. And there is a language problem, which must have been a common occurrence in the days when many Highlanders were not fully bilingual.

Since the patient's Gaelic-speaking wife mistook 'carrots' for 'catechism', a further amusement might be derived from the fact that for such a connection to be made the lady must have pronounced 'carrots' without the normal 'r' sound, or rather she pronounced it according to her own custom of southern speech. The patient's wife, too polite to query the term, might have been utterly baffled had it not been for a memory of the old Gaelic custom of using pages of the scriptures (and the catechism and Bunyan came second best) as a charm against sickness and other evils.

A son of the Dotair Bàn and father of Dr M.D. Macleod was one of many ministers who took his medical sideline seriously. Dr Macleod recalled in 1896, 'I remember when lancets were a part of the equipment of the manse, and my father, till later years, bled his parishioners when he or they thought it beneficial.'

Similarly, the Revd Donald Sage wrote in his *Memorabilia Domestica*, of one of his father's tenants in the Strath of Kildonan, 'Mr Donald Macleod, parochial schoolmaster . . . was very useful in the parish, for he could let blood, and was a daily reader of Buchan's *Domestic Medicine* all whose instructions he rigidly, and often successfully, practised.'[3]

The service that William Buchan, a graduate of the Edinburgh Medical School, rendered to the sick of many rural parishes throughout Britain and overseas, with his excellent *Domestic Medicine* (1769), was recognised not only in his eventual burial in Westminster Abbey, but by the tremendous success of his book. The Faculty of Medicine frowned on his aims to educate ordinary men and women in simple medical methods and rules of health but, to their credit, the ordinary people had the common sense to adopt much of Buchan's advice, which included – again to the scorn of the Faculty – advocation of inoculation against smallpox. Between 1769 and 1826 the book was to run to twenty-two editions, and was as popular in the Highlands as anywhere.

Prior to *Domestic Medicine,* the most popular Scottish book on family medicine was John Moncrief's *Poor Man's Physician* (1712) which advocated such cures as choking and cutting open a 'little black suckling puppy' and extracting 'three or four drops of pure choler' from its gall as a 'miracle cure' for epilepsy in small children. Such practices were a far cry from the simples employed by the Gaels and almost a perversion of the dramatic rituals advised for epileptics. Whatever the idiosyncrasies of traditional Highland medicine, it did not involve cruelty to man's best friend.

The arrival of Buchan's book was, to the domestic medical literature of the time, like the opening of a window on a darkened, stuffy sickroom. His advice for care of health harked back to the best of the guidance in the clan physicians' manuscripts and looked forward to even better ideas. He advocated simple food and exercise, hygiene and sensible clothes, but his most interesting counsels are on the care of children. He advised fathers to take a greater interest in their upbringing and cautioned for little ones to be kept clean with frequent changes of clothing ('Children perspire more than adults . . .'). Buchan was also ever-mindful of the poor and concerned to recommend remedies that were easily available and reasonably cheap. His berating of the unhealthy habits of the better-off may have gone a long way to endearing him to his more needy readers.

8

'AS LONG AS GRASS GROWS'

In April 1818 the Medical Society of the North[1] issued rules for the regulation of doctors' fees, and for this purpose the Highland population was divided into four classes: higher, second, third and fourth. It was a genuine attempt to be fair by charging the rich more and the poor less. 'These regulations', the Society declared, 'are by no means intended to confine the liberality of the higher classes in particular cases, nor to preclude the humanity of the practitioner towards the lower.'

Consultations at the doctor's house were to be charged at one guinea, 10s 6d, 5s, or 2s 6d according to the patient's 'class' which was to be determined by income. Home visits in the town were charged at similar rates (the 10s 6d fee being lowered to 7s 6d) and country visits were charged at two guineas, one guinea and 10s 6d (for third and fourth classes) as well as travelling expenses, chronic cases being charged at half the rate.

Various treatments, such as the dressing of wounds and ulcers, bleeding and teeth-pulling, and minor operations were charged for on top of this. For example, vaccinations cost, respectively, one guinea, 15s, 7s 6d and 5s; attendance at the delivery of a child was ten, five, three, or one guinea(s), with surcharges for night visits. Postnatal visits and consultations with the midwife were extra.[2]

All of this was rather more high-minded than realistic at a time when workers counted their weekly wage in shillings rather than pounds and the very poor received relief (if they were 'deserving') in little more than pennies per week.[3] As with the medical ministrations of the lairds, ministers and dominies, much would depend on the altruism of the individual doctor. Where doctors were to be found at all in the more remote areas, they often had to settle for payment in kind.

Family networks and caring neighbours more often than not helped out with food, a roof and other essentials when people fell on hard times. With doctors' fees being generally beyond the reach of the poor, economic as well as cultural and geographic factors ensured that traditional cures survived in many parts well into the twentieth century. Over and above such basic considerations, the more financially secure who were chronically sick or terminally ill sometimes resorted to traditional healers and remedies in hope of the cure that orthodox medicine was failing to provide, much as people today resort to complementary practitioners.

One example of such a cure occurred in Melness, Sutherland, about a hundred years ago. An army pensioner with a stomach ulcer which city doctors declared incurable, returned from Edinburgh to Melness to seek out an elderly woman relative by the name of Giorsail (Grace) who treated him with infusions made from bogbean, a plant which grows profusely in local moorland pools. He made a full recovery and lived a healthy life for many years.[4]

The breakdown in the old order was to culminate in the enforced clearances of the nineteenth century. The land troubles and poverty of those years remain bitterly engraved in Highland memory. The burning of houses, the laying waste of crops, the wholesale evictions, the scorning of the people's voice[5], created a communal state of trauma that was, for many years, to leach away self-confidence and vitality of spirit. Small wonder that, local employment problems apart, many men opted for a life in the army where a measure of self-esteem might be restored.

Between 1811 and 1820 some 15,000 people were removed from the fertile straths of the north to the inhospitable, windswept and rocky coastline, or to the colonies, to make way for sheep farms. The sad story was repeated throughout the west and the islands involving smaller numbers but even worse acts of inhumanity. Severe climatic deterioration and poor harvests in the wake of a massive volcanic eruption in Iceland in 1783[6], a growing Highland population, agricultural reforms, an underlying boom/bust economic cycle (the main period of Victorian expansion not beginning until around 1840), and perhaps even a concern that the peasantry as well as the urban working classes might be tempted to take a lead from the events of the French Revolution[7], combined to create the atmosphere in which the Clearances were carried out. There were, in the light of nineteenth-century thinking, many good reasons for reforming the economy of the Highlands. There are no excuses for the way in which it was generally carried out.

Throughout the century the people's standards of living, housing and health declined. English, not Gaelic, had become the vehicle for education when the Scottish Society for the Propagation of Christian Knowledge was set up in 1709 and this was reinforced by the Education Act of 1872. Although, from 1811 to 1872, the *Sgoilean Gàidhlig* did splendid work in educating people in their own language, many people's schooling was patchy at best and restricted to primary level, the result being a Gaelic education of sorts and a general failure to achieve the target of fluency in English.

Yet there were still those who kept alive the essence of their culture in the poorest of circumstances. Serious folklore collectors such as John Francis Campbell, John Gregorson Campbell, and Alexander Carmichael were able to amass considerable material despite the encroachment of the southern view of life. Almost all of the cures given in Part II of this book were still being practised somewhere in the Highlands throughout the nineteenth century and a number of them were still in use in the first half of the twentieth, but by a decreasing number of adept healers. As emigration continued, so more and more of the old knowledge seeped away to the colonies and was forgotten at home. Sheep gobbled plants that had once been abundant and the good old days of the summer shielings when the people took to the hills with their cattle and lived almost at one with nature were disappearing. Besides, the old ways could not cope with epidemics, the spread of tuberculosis and the myriad troubles caused by increasing contact with strangers. Orthodox medicine was improving all the time, but few practitioners had ambitions in the Highlands where as late as 1911 a GP might earn as little as £40 a year and be expected to give many of his services for free.

Nevertheless, despite the poverty and uncertainty of those years, the people retained many skills, not least among them the knowledge of home-distilling and brewing. It also seems that in rural areas the problems of drunkenness were not so rife – or at least so obvious – as in the towns and cities, perhaps stemming from a respect for the often greater potency of illicit whisky combined with the hold of the clergy on smaller communities.

In the northern mainland there was a saying to advise on the quantity of whisky that might be drunk at a sitting with safety and, as it was believed, with benefit: *Aona ghloine, chan fheairrde 's cha mhisd'. Dà ghloine 's fheairrde 's cha mhisd'. Trì gloineachan 's misde 's chan fheairrd'.* (One glass, not the better of it or the worse of it. Two glasses, the better of them, and not the worse of them. Three glasses, the worse of them and not the better.) A variation of this was: '*Aon ghloine chan fheairrde 's cha mhisde mo chorp no m'anam e. Dà ghloine, 's fheairrde mo chorp e, 's cha mhisde m'anam e. Trì gloineachan 's misde m'anam e, 's chan fheairrde mo chorp e.*' ('One glass, neither my body nor my soul is the better or the worse of it. Two glasses, my body is the better of them, and my soul is not the worse of them. Three glasses, my soul is the worse for them, and my body is not the better of them.')

As medicinal drugs, beers and spirits had few rivals for esteem. 'May the Lord preserve us from the disease whisky cannot cure!' ran a popular Highland saying, and virtually every community had access to the products of illicit stills. Katherine Whyte Grant, whose information given to the Caledonian Medical Society in 1904 is an invaluable source of late nineteenth-century cures, relates that whisky, often known euphemistically as 'heather ale' or 'mountain dew', was one of the great specifics: 'There was generally on hand a supply of home-made stuff and, failing that, those who had no still could in a time of extremity make shift to brew it with the help of the kettle – I know *my* grandmother could.'[8]

Diarrhoea, which did not respond to other treatment, was said to be instantly cured by setting a match to a glassful of whisky which was allowed to flame for two or three minutes. When extinguished, the whisky had to be drunk right away.

A mixture of whisky and sulphur was given to a patient in order to 'get the measles' rash out'. But whisky was not the only spirit employed, rum was also popular, especially in areas where the men were seafarers. An understandably popular cure for a persistent cough was to take a glass of beer added to one of rum two or three times a day.

Bloodletting continued to be practised in some areas until as late as the 1930s, and was often carried out by blacksmiths, perhaps the last vestige of their ancient connections with healing.

On the north coast of Sutherland it was claimed that Murdo Macpherson of Melness who died around 1880 was 'bred from Fearchar (Lighiche)'s breed'. Murdo used the horse leech, *gearrach-dall*, to bleed people with fevers. His son Donald lived to the ripe age of ninety-three (another son, Robert, lived to be ninety-seven), and claimed that his longevity was due to never having put salt on his food. No salt was used in cooking by the family. 'If anyone wanted salt they'd add it later at table,' Hugh Macdonald, of Skinnet, told me. Long walks every day were another of this family's prescriptions for a healthy life. Such practices are certainly reminiscent of the advice given by the Beatons.

The alarm spread by the activities of the notorious body-snatchers Burke and Hare and others had its repercussions well beyond urban

Scotland. In the early decades of the nineteenth century the facilities for acquiring anatomical and pathological knowledge were very limited, and it is beyond doubt that cases of 'premature resurrection', as Dr James Logan of the Caledonian Medical Society put it, did occasionally take place. There is also no doubt that the popular imagination could magnify and distort the extent of gruesome practice. Legends abounded. Logan recounted to his colleagues that he had often heard of the 'wild' or 'black' doctors, a fearful brotherhood, whose great object was to obtain human bodies, and who 'scrupled not to take away life for their own evil ends'. Their feared weapon was the *black patch* – a highly adhesive plaster which, when suddenly applied over the mouth and nose, stopped all cries, and produced speedy suffocation. The feeing market at Inverness was said to be a special hunting-ground for luring country girls to a dreadful fate, doubtless before as well as after death. Thus far the stories might be credible, but the public imagination added a truly inventive rider. The object of the 'black doctors', it was claimed, was not anatomical, but pharmaceutical: the bodies being boiled down yielding a broth of such marvellous healing quality that people who were wasted with disease and racked with pain were speedily restored to perfect health and comfort by its use. Dr Logan added: 'I also heard it hinted that this terrible process was the source of castor oil!'

People who lived through that Highland era of dispossession and uncertainty might be excused for believing that such horrors were likely. But by 1854 attitudes had begun to harden. In that year the Sutherland men of the 93rd Regiment were ordered to the Crimea where they were to achieve enduring fame as the 'thin red line tipped with steel' at Balaclava. The regiment was renowned for its discipline, military skills and courage and those who fought at Balaclava were seasoned fighters – to a man. Not one new recruit from the younger men of the Duke of Sutherland's estates had been persuaded to enlist after Britain declared war on Russia. 'We have no country to fight for. You robbed us of our country and gave it to the sheep. Therefore, since you have preferred sheep to men, let sheep defend you,' the recruiting agents were told.

Shortly before the 93rd departed for the Crimea in September 1854, the able-bodied men who refused to enlist drew up a public statement justifying their case:

> We have no country to fight for, as our glens and straths are laid desolate, and we have no wives nor children to defend as we are forbidden to have them. We are not allowed to marry without the consent of the factor, the ground officer being always ready to report every case of marriage, and the result would be banishment from the county. Our lands have been taken from us and given to sheep farmers, and we are denied any portion of them, and when we apply for such, or even a site for a house, we are told that we should leave the country. For these wrongs and oppressions, as well as for others which we have long and patiently endured, we are resolved that there shall be no volunteers or recruits from Sutherlandshire. Yet we assert that we are as willing as our forefathers were to peril life and limb in defence of our Queen and country were our wrongs and long-endured oppression redressed, wrongs which will be remembered in Sutherlandshire by every true Highlander as long as grass grows and water runs.[9]

The movement for security of land tenure was to gather momentum, and, although all was not won, a significant victory was achieved in the Crofting Act of 1886. Recruitment to the Highland regiments, however, became yet again a matter for concern by the beginning of the twentieth century, but for rather different reasons.

Work was never easy to come by in the new Highlands of the vast sporting estates which, by the mid-nineteenth century, had taken over from the sheep farms as the main land use. Crofting, limited to tenancies of a very few acres of marginal agricultural land, and in some places mere rock-strewn coastal strips, was never designed to be anything more than a part-time activity. Those men who could not, or would not, find employment with the laird rarely had other than three options, outright emigration, work away from home (with rare visits to their families), or enlistment in the army or navy. The last course was welcomed by the government.

There was, however, a problem. While there were now men keen to join the army, all too many had to be turned down on health grounds. It was the continuing need to recruit soldiers, fortified by memories of the land unrest of the late nineteenth century and pressure from Highland Members of Parliament, that forced Westminster into finding a solution to deteriorating standards of health. In 1911 a committee was appointed under the chairmanship of Sir John Dewar, MP for Inverness-shire, 'to consider at an early date how far the provision of medical attendance in [the Highlands and Islands] is adequate, and to advise as to the best method of securing a satisfactory medical service therein . . .'

The Dewar report[10] on health and medical services in the Highlands and Islands which was completed by the following year remains an extraordinary social document, rivalled in the Highlands only by the Napier Commission's exhaustive inquiries into crofting conditions three decades earlier. Where the Napier report was to result in the Crofting Act, the Dewar one was eventually to have even further-reaching consequences for the whole United Kingdom. Lloyd George's National Health Insurance Scheme of 1911 was acknowledged to be unworkable in the small scattered communities of north-west Scotland where the people subsisted on scant and irregular incomes. What was to be done?

The Dewar committee, which toured the area and obtained first-hand evidence from over 250 witnesses (including more than ninety doctors and a number of crofters, teachers, ministers, and fishermen), reported that, with honourable exceptions, the quality of medical and nursing care was poor, and the coverage very fragmented. The combination of social, economic and geographical difficulties in the Highlands demanded exceptional treatment.

Within eight months of the publication of the report an Act of Parliament established the Highlands and Islands Medical Service Fund 'for improving medical services, including nursing, in the Highlands and Islands of Scotland, and otherwise providing and improving means for the prevention, treatment and alleviation of illness and suffering therein'.

Money was made available from central government to make up or cover doctors' and nurses' salaries, surgery equipment and housing, specialist, hospital and ambulance services, and telegraph and telephone services. It was to anticipate the National Health Service by over thirty-five years, although until that full service came in, in 1948, small agreed fees (of 5s for the first visit, 2s 6d for subsequent visits in the same illness and £1 for midwifery cases) were payable by even the very lowest income groups.

The project was revolutionary in its concept and so successful in its application that by 1947 the chief medical officer of the Department of Health for Scotland could confidently say:

> We have no difficulty in obtaining doctors, specialists or nurses for any area within the scheme; indeed the numbers and calibre of applicants for vacancies are frequently embarrassing.[11]

Many of those same doctors, specialists and nurses were the sons and daughters of Highland crofts, manses, schoolhouses where the often fragile threads of an old culture with its enduring love of learning and inquiry and tradition of community caring were beginning to interweave with some intriguing and robust new colours.

9

A FUTURE FOR THE PAST?

Something I have continually asked myself while looking back into the story of the Gaelic medical tradition is whether some part of it has a future beyond antiquarian rummaging in its intricacies. Might not some of its cures, and something of its philosophy be worthy of investigation by people qualified in medicine and pharmaceutics? If twenty remedies were to be investigated and only one found to be of any value in modern medicine, surely it would be worth the trouble?

The talks I have given in villages and towns throughout the Highlands and Islands over recent years have almost always been attended by the local GP and, where there was one, the pharmacist. Far from being dismissive they turned out to be the most attentive and supportive members of the audience. Many were fascinated by and agreed with the common sense of the most psychologically influenced cures. Almost all were able to contribute reasons as to how certain remedies may have worked; some were able to shed considerable light on methods that may have seemed quite bizarre to lay listeners; and they often came up with parallels in modern medicine.

In 1977 the World Health Organisation initiated a scheme, involving numerous governments and international institutions, to seek out and examine local remedies in remote parts of the globe – and the exercise has brought many benefits.[1] Not only has the knowledge of traditional healers in, for instance, the Brazilian Rain Forest been accorded a growing respect but some of their cures, especially the herbal ones, are proving valuable in Western medicine. It has also given these remote (to us) people a renewed sense of their own worth.

Yet here on the fringes of Western Europe we have – in hitherto largely untapped manuscript, documentary and personal sources – a huge body of traditional medical knowledge which is surely worthy of professional investigation. Not all these cures were necessarily efficient – many have rightly been superseded by far better modern drugs and techniques – and no one in their right mind would wish to return to medieval standards of surgery and dental care, but a case can be made for having a closer, scientific look at our native lore. Has anyone yet investigated the possible therapeutic uses of slug and snail slime, which is easily acquired and need incur no rebuke from a Gasteropods' Rights lobby, for skin growths, or does its employment in folk medicine (see Chapter 12) smack too much of the altogether 'quaint'? The recipe given in Chapter 12 for the nourishing jelly made from naturally shed antlers deserves to be better known and used in convalescent diets.

Highland herbal lore includes uses of some plants not, to my knowledge, even taken account of in modern herbal wisdom. Take, for example, the tuberous vetch – the discussion of it in Chapter 14 suggests it may have some uses in the treatment of alcohol, nicotine or diet-related problems.

Since the skill of the former healers has virtually disappeared, it would be foolish for the half-taught to tinker with such remedies as those derived from St John's Wort. The injudicious use of this herb can have harmful side-effects, especially those stemming from its capacity for increasing photo-sensitivity which might lead to skin cancers and other problems. The queen of the meadow, or meadowsweet, would probably also need expert investigation, but there may be a future for it in headache remedies. It was once widely used among the Gaels for such problems and may even owe some of its healing property to its aroma alone. I have noticed myself that the head clears wonderfully after a walk through the plants, but there is a better story.

A doctor's wife who is herself a qualified nurse told me how for months she had been plagued by persistent headaches which nothing would shift with any lasting effect. Then one day the pains simply vanished for good, just how she could not tell. It was my mention of the meadowsweet and its properties during a talk in her local primary school hall that prompted her to remember. The day the headaches left her she had, for the first time, picked a huge bunch of the flowers and put them in the house where their pervasive scent lingered for days. Now, there is nothing very scientific about that anecdote but surely enough of a hint to provoke deeper investigation.

The list might go on: the bogbean for stomach upsets and ulcers; herb Robert for skin treatments; wild carrot for certain cancers; heather for the nerves; pink centaury as a tonic; honeysuckle for chestiness; and seaweeds for a variety of conditions.

The present call for diversification in agriculture might be satisfied in some small part by the occasional plot of land being devoted to homegrown plants for the pharmaceutical industry, as indeed occurs in other parts of the world, e.g. the Scottish Crop Research Institute is currently promoting the advantages of sea buckthorn (a shrub which thrives on poor windswept soils) as a commercial crop with high value for the food, cosmetics, soft drinks and pharmaceutical industries. Long known as a useful plant in Chinese medicine, it is now being grown commercially both there and in Russia. The blaeberry was a valued healing plant in the Highlands and there might be great possibilities for its remedial use in this country.

While medicine must always look to advancing its theories and practice for the greater betterment of humanity, it can surely do no harm to turn a fresh eye on old methods that may have been discarded for no better reason than that they had fallen out of fashion.

In her novel *Silas Marner* in which she so splendidly captures the passing of an old village way of life in the mid-nineteenth century, George Eliot writes:

Silas sat down now and watched Eppie with a satisfied gaze as she spread the clean cloth, and set on it the potato pie, warmed up slowly in a safe Sunday fashion, by being put into a dry pot over a slowly-dying fire, as the best substitute for an oven. For Silas would not consent to have a grate and oven added to his conveniences: he loved the old brick hearth as he had loved his brown pot – and was it not there when he found Eppie? The gods of the hearth exist for us still; and let all new faith be tolerant of that fetishism, lest it bruise its own roots.[2]

There in a distinctively English story we have a universal problem of peculiar relevance in a Highland setting. Few but romantically minded incomers would now look at anything but a modern cooker, but there remains a strong wariness of bruising old roots. A story told of Calum Cille says that when he was founding his church in Derry (named after the Gaelic for oak wood) he was unhappy about having the sacred trees of the old druidic grove felled in order to clear land for his chapel. To get round this, the building was made to face north rather than, as is traditional in Christianity, towards the east. Later in life, he admitted that 'though he feared Death and Hell, the sound of an axe in the grove of Derry frightened him still more'. From what is known of Calum Cille's austere attitude to superstition, it may be taken that he was fearful not so much of vengeful spirits as of breaking the sense of continuity that was so important to his people's way of life. New ideas, both Eliot and Calum Cille are saying, must form part of a natural progression.

The sequence may also work in reverse. In looking back on the old roots of the healing 'tree' we must not ignore the new leaves and shoots. It hardens sceptical professional attitudes only when un-critical nostalgia is shown for some golden-green harmony of ancient herbalism. Orthodox medicine is becoming increasingly aware of the benefits that may be gained from taking account of traditional methods, it would be good to see more of complementary medicine seeing the real values of modern science. Best of all, much might be achieved when the two can work in full accord – with just a touch of rivalry to spur yet further investigations and keep them all on their toes.

Chemically created formulae can make use of animal healing properties without harming live creatures as the old remedies did. Plant extracts can be made into regulated doses where natural herbs may vary considerably in the strength of their remedial (or, indeed, toxic) components. Although an argument may be made for the possibly beneficial balance of differing constituents in one plant as opposed to the extraction of one element, surely the way forward is, again, by collaboration.

Both strains of modern outlook might gain by the prime qualities of the best of the old Gaelic healers, their innate common sense and their spirit of inquiry, and their uncanny understanding of the psychological and spiritual needs of the patient.

Now we have what they lacked: technology and a wider grasp of the workings of mind and body. If only a modicum of their knowledge turns out to be worthy of serious respect by present day science, then the search may prove as valuable as the outcome in providing us with a touch of those more elusive qualities — wisdom and understanding.

Alongside all the cures there has been one unwavering thread of strength, the Gaelic language. Its terms for diseases are concerned more with the way patients experience the problem than from detached observation of the condition. *Greim fala* or *teaghaid*, for instance, are two terms for pleurisy and refer to the sharp, spear-like thrust of the acute pain actually suffered, rather than the condition of the lung. The vivid diagnostic vocabulary leaves patients in no doubt that the physician knows exactly how they are suffering. The language as a whole, with its rhythms, perceptions, its strangely subtle precision and its descriptive genius might have been custom-made for the doctor/patient relationship. A society for the promotion of Gaelic in health care in the relevant areas of the Highlands and islands was formed in 1992. While the immediate aim of *Comann Gàidhlig Seirbheis na Slàinte* – founded by a group of doctors, nurses, paramedics and other health service employees – is to benefit Gaelic-speaking patients, its belief in the use of familiar language and helpful communication has wider-reaching implications.

The following grace said by Farquhar Beaton, who lived from about 1750 to 1850, was once known in Skye as *Urnaigh a'Pheutanaich*, Beaton's Prayer. It seems as good a wish for the way forward as any, and it bruises no roots. The modern mind might prefer to substitute 'vain illusions' for the 'dominion of fairies' and 'envy' for 'evil eye'. An older society preferred to express the intangible in concrete forms. Whether we cope any better by intellectualising that unease is another question.

O Thì bheannaichte, cùm ruinn, agus cuidich leinn, agus na tuiteadh do ghràs oirnn mar an t-uisge air druim a' gheòidh. An uair a bhios fear 'na éiginn air gob rubha, cuidich féin leis; agus bi mun cuairt duinn air tìr, agus maille ruinn. Gléidh an t-aosda agus an t-òga, ar mnathan agus ar pàisdean, ar spréidh agus ar feudal, o chumhachd agus o cheannas nan sithichean, agus o mhì-rùn gach droch shùla. Bitheadh slighe réidh romhainn, agus crìoch shona air ar turas.

O Blessed One, provide for us, and help us, and let not thy grace fall on us like the rain on the goose's back. When a man is in danger on the point of a promontory, do thou succour him; and be about us on land, and with us. Preserve the old and the young, our wives and our children, our sheep and our cattle, from the power and from the dominion of the fairies, and from the malice of every evil eye. Let a smooth path be before us, and a happy end to our journey.

MATERIA MEDICA

10

WATERS, WELLS AND
HEALING SPRINGS

The oldest place-names tend to be the names of rivers.[1] It might be argued whether rivers were named after deities, usually female, or vice versa, but at the time of the naming the two probably shared the same 'personality'. In such a way, healing wells and springs, too, would have come to have their own identity. When they began to be recorded in the Middle Ages, most had acquired an association with a Christian saint. Dedicated to goddess or saint, the successive traditions were probably simply a way of embodying the 'spirit' or feeling engendered by the site or influenced by its setting in the landscape, or the peculiar quality of its waters.

The origin of distinct sites for the healing of specific diseases or the performance of remedial rituals occurred before written history. Some water was notorious for harming rather than healing, but this only added to the wonder engendered by this most rudimentary of substances. It is also true that some of the most remedial waters, such as sulphur springs, are disagreeable to taste which makes early researches into their value all the more praiseworthy. What is probably the earliest Highland record of a people awestruck by a spring occurs in Adomnán's Life of Columba:

> At one time, when the blessed man passed some days in the province of the Picts, he heard that the fame of [a] well was widespread among

the heathen populace, and that the insensate people venerated it as a god, the devil deluding their understanding. For those that drank from this well, or deliberately washed their hands or feet in it, were struck, by devilish art, God permitting it, and returned leprous, or half blind, or even crippled, or suffering from some other infirmity. Led astray by all this, the heathen gave honour to the well as to a god. When he learned of that, the saint went boldly to the well one day. The magicians, whom he often repelled from himself in confusion and defeat, rejoiced greatly when they saw this, since they imagined that he would suffer the like ills, from touching that noxious water. But he, first raising his holy hand in invocation of the name of Christ, washed his hands and feet; and after that, with those that accompanied him, drank of the same water, which he had blessed. And from that day, the demons withdrew from that well, and not only was it not permitted to harm any one, but after the saint's blessing, and washing in it, many infirmities among the people were in fact cured by the same well.[2]

Under various headings below are listed examples of the diverse uses of water and the places associated with them.

'ANNAT WELLS' or BURNS (G. *annaid*)

These healing wells or streams are always situated close to the site of a small early church, chapel or cemetery, most of which are now mere ruins if visible at all. The word occurs in numerous place-names, e.g. na h-Annaidean (Shader, Lewis); Achadh na h-Annaide (the Field of the Annat), in a number of districts; Clach na h-Annaide (the Stone of the Annat), in Strathconon; Tobar na h-Annaide (the Well of the Annat), at Kilbride in Skye, and so forth.

By association with a particular saint or church, and probably even earlier pagan deities, peculiar virtues were attributed to the waters. Otherwise these usually remote sites seem to have been unimportant. Some such waters may simply have been so named because of their drinking quality. In his great poem *Moladh Beinn Dobhrain* (the Praise of

Ben Dorain) composed some time during the years 1751–66, Duncan
Bàn Macintyre says:

> Fìon uillt na h-Annaid,
> Blas meala r' a òl air.
> (The wine of the burn of the Annat,
> Honey-flavoured to drink.)

This stream, which runs into the Conghlais river at the foot of Ben
Dorain, also gave *ìocshlainte mhaireann*, enduring healing. The last
known cure at the well of Annat near the head of Loch Torridon in
Wester Ross occurred within living memory. A man suffering from
epilepsy undertook the ancient regime of drinking the well water from
a suicide's skull every sunrise and sunset for two weeks. Then he was
put under a *geas*, injunction, not to drink to excess or to go under a
bier (carry a coffin to the cemetery). The cure, which probably owed
not a little to the stricture on alcohol, was said to have been highly
successful and the man lived a healthy life for many years. The well is
said to have lost its efficacy through a shepherd having taken his dog
to drink at it.

BAPTISMAL WATER

Water used for a baptism was carefully bottled and kept as a cure
for any sicknesses the infant might encounter. In line with the old
Gaelic interest in preventive medicine, a baptised infant was neither
washed nor bathed on the night following the ceremony, for fear
of washing off the baptismal water before it had slept under it. It
was believed that if the 'holy water' was washed off the child would
never thrive.

CAVES

Caves, and especially the water found in them, had a particular
significance. The dripping cave of Craig-a-Chowie on the Black Isle

was resorted to for the cure of earache and deafness. The patient was held so as to let a drop of the cave-water fall into the afflicted ear. Under the main drip of water there is a stone, coloured a deep red, as if stained. The story goes that long ago a mother took her baby, who had been born deaf, with her to be healed. As the drop fell into the ear, the infant screamed and wriggled. '*Sgàin* [burst]!' exclaimed the mother, impatiently. The imprecation, so the story goes, took effect, and the blood of the infant dyed the stone.

It was once believed that fairies lived in the cave and carried off the cattle that strayed into it. Two children, a boy and a girl, wandered in and were never again seen. Such tales are commonly connected with caves and probably originated as deterrents to children who might be tempted to venture into potentially dangerous areas. By 1900 the entrance to the Craig-a-Chowie cavern was blocked off, as one report had it, 'to prevent all accident to man or beast'. For the same reason this was done to numerous caves and underground caverns, including man-made souterrains, throughout the Highlands, especially after sheep were introduced.

CHALYBEATE SPRINGS

These iron-rich springs were much visited, especially in mild cases of tuberculosis. Such springs were popular throughout the country. At Hart Fell spa, 1200 feet high on the Auchencat Burn, four miles north of Moffat in Dumfriesshire, the chalybeate waters were once believed to be particularly beneficial for women's complaints. I have not been able to discover, so far, whether such springs were used specifically for the same purpose in the Highland tradition but iron-bearing water would certainly make sense for the anaemia-related ills to which a number of women are prone.

A glance at detailed Ordnance Survey maps for the Highlands will show an abundance of chalybeate springs and many of them were once resorted to for cures or simply drinking water. Four such springs at

Pannanich, near Ballater, were famed for curing many diseases, most notably scrofula.[3]

COLD OR HOT WATER?

In some cures the temperature of the water was important and there might be specific instructions for using either cold or hot water. People with scrofula, for example, were advised to expose the afflicted part every day to a stream of cold water, whereas urinary obstructions were relieved by taking a hot bath.

Good simple advice for clearing up pimples on the face was to drink plenty of cold water until the spots vanished. When modern remedies for pneumonia failed, the old practice of putting the patient in a tub of hot water was said to be effective.

EVIL EYE

Beliefs about the phenomenon called the evil eye – in Gaelic, the *droch shùil* or *buidseachd* – were much the same in Highland tradition as elsewhere in the world, the possessor of the 'eye' being generally accepted as not necessarily *consciously* responsible for any ill befalling the victim. As in other cultures, the occurrence was believed to stem from jealousy, therefore those who incurred the 'evil' might be considered to have brought it on themselves by in some way inciting envy or resentment. A strong conviction in cause and effect lay behind the belief that the evil eye was responsible for a run of bad luck, when no more mundane reason could be found. But 'antidotes' were plentiful, and among them water played its part.

Certain preparations of water, in which gold, silver and copper – usually coins or rings – were placed, formed the basis of the cure. If possible, the water was to be fetched from a place 'where the living and dead passed by', that is near or under a bridge which served as a common path both for daily travel and the route on which coffins were carried to the churchyard. The cure consisted in sprinkling a few handfuls of the water on the affected person or animal with the usual invocation of the Trinity (see Chapter 13, Rituals, Charms and Incantations). The remainder was either poured on the fire, or taken outside and spilled on a rock in front of the house.

In Strathhalladale, Sutherland, and elsewhere, the cure was extended to humans and beasts believed to be suffering not only from the evil eye but from any 'witchcraft' spell. Here the water was given to the victim to drink.

Sometimes water from a very special spring might be used without adding gold and silver. The water from Fuaran Dheòradh (Spring of the Afflicted) was in great demand for curing bewitched animals in the Durness area.

LOCHS

Loch Mo Nàire, in Strathnaver, was famous throughout the north for its healing water which, for the best effect, was supposed to be used on the first Monday of a quarter, the May and August ones being the most popular, no doubt because the climate was warmer. The majority of patients came from the neighbouring county of Caithness, but many also flocked from other parts of Sutherland, Ross-shire, Inverness-shire and Orkney, since there was a belief that a more certain cure was to be had from waters outside one's own parish. Invalids arrived the day before taking the cure and were kept tied up and fed sparingly until sunset. At around midnight they were unbound and assembled near the loch where they were stripped naked. As the first streak of the early northern summer dawn appeared their attendants directed them to walk backwards into the dark, cold waters of the loch until they were fully immersed. As this was being done coins were thrown into the water. The patients were then pulled out, dressed in silence and walked sunwise around the loch's edge. Then they had to walk away without once turning their heads, until they were out of sight of the water before the sun rose.

Many of the people who underwent this stringent ritual were suffering from some form of mental disease in varying degrees of severity from mild depression to outright mania, so it seems reasonable to suppose that the sheer drama of the setting and events, and the trauma of the immersion must have acted as a form of shock treatment. Certainly the enduring popularity of the proceedings must bear some witness to at least occasional cures. Coachloads of people from Caithness still visited the loch at least until the late 1930s.

Several lochs have associations with healing legends but rather more because of the rituals conducted on or near them than because of the virtue of the water itself. Loch Maree in Wester Ross is a prime example, but since a well on one of its small islands was central to the cure, the story will be given under **WELLS** (below) as will that of the small St Fillan's Loch. A cure for asthma related to me in Glenmoriston, Inverness-shire, in 1958, involved rising well before dawn and rowing a boat, alone, across the loch. The return journey had to be completed before the sun rose.

SEA

For *leamhnad*, a stye, standing on the head in the sea until nine waves pass over you, or counting one hundred without drawing breath, was considered effectual. The salt water may well have been beneficial, but there are easier ways of applying it.

The archives of the School of Scottish Studies, University of Edinburgh, have a record of a Tiree remedy (in a cutting from the North British Mail of 20 March, 1883) for jaundice which involved boiling nine stones in water taken from the crests of nine waves. The patient's shirt was dipped in this infusion and put on wet. An alternative was to take water from nine springs or streams in which cresses grow.

A popular cure for a bad cold was for the patient to be immersed, fully clad, in the sea, then to run straight home and go to bed, still in the wet clothing, and sleep off the ailment. More gentle bathing in sea water was resorted to for certain bone diseases and rheumatism, at the same time drinking a cup of the brine. Sea water also made a free and effective purgative.

STRATHPEFFER

This was a popular Highland spa, attracting visitors from all over after its powers were widely advertised in 1819. In the seventeenth century, the famous Mackenzie seer, Coinneach Odhar, is said to have foretold of Strathpeffer: 'Uninviting and disagreeable as it is now, with its thick crusted surface and unpleasant smell, the day will come when it shall be under lock and key, and crowds of pleasure- and health-seekers shall be seen thronging its portals, in their eagerness to get a draught of its waters.' These waters are said to contain more sulphurated hydrogen than any in Britain, and while there are many other minerals present, it is for the strength of sulphur in its water that Strathpeffer is most famous. The Old Well, the Duchess of Sutherland's Well, Dr Morrison's Well and the Countess of Cromartie's Well are all sulphur springs, while the Iron Well is, as its name confirms, a chalybeate one.

SWEATING CURES

In common with the Scandinavians and native Americans, the Gaels of Ireland and Scotland were great ones for sweating cures and steam baths, and it is possible that what archaeologists call 'burnt mound sites' may sometimes be the remains of old sweathouses. Sites can vary in date from anything between the Bronze Age and late medieval times, and also in size, but basically they consist of a mass of burnt stones frequently accompanied by a sunken flagstone-lined pit or tank. In Scotland well over 800 such sites have been recorded and more are being discovered all the time. Several arguments have been put forward as to their use, but it is beyond dispute that the burnt stones had been heated in fires and plunged into the tanks – or other receptacles – in order to heat water.

The archaeologist, John Barber, has said: 'Boiling water has many uses, and while cooking may be the most common of them it is certainly not the only one. There is no reason not to assume that some burnt mounds were used for bathing, washing, saunas, sweathouses and a range of semi-industrial functions of which we have as yet little indication.'[4]

The appearance of quartz pebbles in a number of these sites begs an analogy with Martin Martin's description of a sweating cure used in Skye at the end of the seventeenth century:

> The antient way the Islanders us'd to procure Sweat, was thus: A part of an earthen Floor was cover'd with Fire, and when it was sufficiently heated, the Fire was taken away, and the ground cover'd with a Heap of Straw; upon this Straw a Quantity of Water was poured, and the Patient lying on the Straw; the Heat of it put his whole Body into a sweat. To cause any particular Part of the Body to sweat, they dig an hole in an earthen Floor, and fill it with Hazle Sticks, and dry Rushes; above these they put a Hectick-Stone [quartz] red hot, and pouring some Water in the Hole, the Patient holds the Part affected over it, and this procures a speedy Sweat.[5]

Similar cures were recorded in the Highland mainland towards the end of the nineteenth century by the Caledonian Medical Society. Sweating cures for colds and influenza were particularly common – and often effective provided the patient was carefully tended.

TOOTHACHE

Resorting to holy wells was a favoured relief for toothache, while others believed in baking an oatmeal bannock with saliva, and placing it in water under a bridge where the living and dead cross. As the bannock melted and disappeared, so, too, would the toothache. But the whole procedure had to be carried out in complete silence – if one word or murmur were uttered, all would be in vain.

WELLS

Healing wells occur throughout Scotland, as indeed they do throughout Britain and Ireland, and the stories attached to them have been amply documented. But they had a fascination for the Caledonian Medical Society whose own records contain information not necessarily published elsewhere. The Society's *Journal* contains material on healing wells submitted by Dr S Rutherford MacPhail, Dr Duncan Macgregor and Mrs Katherine Whyte Grant which form the basis of the following accounts. MacPhail, being a Wester Ross man, was well placed to add local knowledge to stories about the famed healing isle in Loch Maree, First, some background detail, beginning with a description of the island given by Thomas Pennant, who visited Innis Maree in 1772:

> The shores are neat and gravelly; the whole surface covered thickly with a beautiful grove of oak, ash, willow, wicken, birch, fir, hazel, and enormous hollies. In the midst is a circular dike of stones, with a regular narrow entrance, the inner part has been used for ages as a burial-place, and is still in use . . . A stump of a tree is shown as an altar, probably the memorial of one stone; but the curiosity of the place is the well of the saint; of power unspeakable in cases of lunacy.[6]

Saint Maelrubha (roughly pronounced Molrua, or Maruya), to whom the well is dedicated, and after whom the island and loch are named, is said to have come to Scotland from Ireland in about 671. After missionary work for the Celtic Church in the north-west Highlands, he settled in the Applecross area which remained his base until he died in 722 at the age of eighty. But in the same area an old Celtic god by the name of Mourie was said to be revered until at least the end of the seventeenth century; and Mourie is an alternative, anglicised, spelling of Maelrubha. The question of Maelrubha/Mourie may well be a male equivalent of the goddess/saint Brigid syndrome. The story told in Chapter 6 of the bulls sacrificed to Mourie on Innis Maree in 1656 and 1678 probably refers to a very ancient practice indeed. In earlier times healing rituals at the well were also accompanied by milk being poured on the ground. The meat of the ritually slaughtered bulls was traditionally given to a class of privileged mendicants called *deirbhleinean Ma-Ruibhe*, Maelrubha's poor ones.

Cloth 'offerings' were hung on branches, or coins were pressed edgeways into the trunks of trees, especially that of an ancient oak growing near the well. On a visit to Loch Maree, Queen Victoria added a coin of her own to the wishing-oak. Rutherford MacPhail told his colleagues in the Caledonian Medical Society how, when his father was a pupil at Ullapool (which must have been well before 1850), one of the bigger boys at the school became mentally deranged:

> His friends took him away by boat to the famous island with its well of virtues in Loch Maree. He was put into the well, and afterwards tied with a rope from the boat and towed round the island three times, but all to no purpose, for he [MacPhail senior] says he can remember vividly the boys waiting on the shore for the return of the boat, expecting to find their schoolfellow all right, but there he was, bound hand and foot, and still a raving maniac.[7]

How many successes and how many failures such procedures generated, it is impossible to say, but nothing seemed to dent the esteem in which such methods were held. Presumably it always helped to sort out what were seen as the malingerers and the poseurs from the genuine cases (although, in its own right, such behaviour is also usually indicative of problems), and may sometimes have worked as shock treatment for certain mental conditions. The fame of Innis

Maree for healing epilepsy, where the patient drank the well water from the skull of a suicide, may have owed something to the sense of drama that was created. St Fillan's chapel and pool in Strathfillan, west Perthshire, was notable for particularly rigorous methods of healing, combining many of the individual cures of other places in, as it were, a gala production. However, it is necessary to disentangle the rituals connected with this site and others relating to St Fillans at the eastern end of Loch Earn, and the St Fillan's *Day* practices at Killin at the south-west end of Loch Tay. In the past several writers appear – easily enough – to have confused the three places which are within around twenty miles of each other. Killin is dealt with under 'Votive Offerings' in Chapter 11; the Loch Earn 'Holy Pool', at the foot of Dùn Fhaolain (Fillan's hill or hillfort), was especially resorted to by barren women and people suffering from rheumatism; St Fillans in Strathfillan was primarily for the cure of insanity. Given the customary kindness with which the congenitally retarded were treated throughout Gaeldom, one can only assume that the families and carers of the patients whose lot is described here by Dr Duncan Macgregor of the Caledonian Medical Society, were themselves at their wits' end:

> The lunatics were first plunged into the water, wherein they were tumbled and tossed about rather roughly. They were then carried into the adjacent chapel of St Fillan's, and there secured with ropes, tied in a special way. A celebrated bell, which has a history of its own, was then placed with great solemnity on the patient's head. There the poor creature was left all night alone in the dreary chapel, and if, in the morning, he was found unloosed, hopes were entertained that he would recover his reason, but the case was hopeless if found still in his bonds. Very frequently the patients were released from their bonds and torments by death, caused by the cold and all the cruelties inflicted on them.[8]

Adding further details to Macgregor's account, Dr MacPhail reported that in early August 1798 an English traveller had recorded in his diary that the holy loch was visited by crowds of people towards the end of the moon's first quarter. Men bathed on one side of a rocky promontory, and women on the other. Each person then took nine stones from the loch and walked to a nearby hill where they did three turns round each of three cairns, leaving a stone each time. In addition, parts of clothing which covered any physical pains or sores were also deposited. If the cure was sought on behalf of a sick animal, some of its meal was brought, made into a paste with water from the loch and later fed to the beast. In order for this cure to be 'infallible', the animal's halter had to be thrown on a cairn. 'Consequently,' noted the traveller, 'the cairns are covered with old halters, gloves, shoes, bonnets, nightcaps, rags of all sorts, kilts, garters, etc.' MacPhail added that mad people were thrown in the water with a rope tied round the middle. At St Fillan's church they were put in a large hollowed stone and fastened into a wooden framework before being left for the night with a covering of hay and the bell itself as a 'nightcap'.[9]

The Black Isle has several healing wells of which the best known are the Dripping Well in the Craig-a-Chowie cave, mentioned above, the Fiddler's Well near Cromarty, once famed for curing consumption, the Craigie Well just above the high-water mark on the north side of Munlochy Bay, and the popularly named Clootie Well on the roadside near Munlochy village itself. Some wells are hard to find, but if you are driving along the A832 from, say, Muir of Ord to Avoch, the Clootie one is impossible to ignore. Bushes on either side of it are heavily festooned with clooties, or wee rags, of all kinds. If you stop and take a closer look, these bits of cloth vary in age from the positively mouldering and decaying to yesterday's fresh offering. Indeed, there are some, perhaps those lately come to the area, who regard it as an 'eyesore', but local tradition will brook no interference.

Unlike many similar sites, the Munlochy Clootie Well – recorded in some books as St Boniface Well – does not carry the custom of having to be visited on a special day (usually before sunrise on 1 May), although this may once have been the case. Anyone might drink of its waters at any time for the help of any disease or the grant of any wish. Traditionally the pieces of thread or cloth left behind should have been somehow related to the part of the body causing a problem but few people are so particular these days. Locals almost anywhere will tell you that it is only the tourists who show an interest in the old customs now. But local people often do keep to the old ways, they are just a bit more discreet.

A friend of mine who lives near the Clootie Well told me how he watched a group of giggling young girls, whose unmistakeable Easter Ross accents carried well enough in the morning air, drinking from the water there. Before they left on their bicycles, they hung their offerings on the bushes. Intrigued by what they might be, my friend waited till the girls were out of sight and went to look. He was not a little abashed at what they had left – some dainty pairs of knickers. Well, why not?

The most remote healing well in Scotland must be Tobar nam Buadh (the Well of the Special Powers) in St Kilda. More latterly its water was supposed to cure deafness and nervous diseases and there was once a nearby altar where prayers were offered. The well is still protected by large stones and was in use until the evacuation of the island in 1930. Martin wrote in his *A Voyage to St Kilda, 1697*:

> I drank of it twice, an English Quart each time; it was very clear, exceeding cold, light and diuretic; I was not able to hold my Hand in it above a few minutes for its Coldness; the Inhabitants of Harries find it effectual against Windy-Cholics, Gravel, and Head-aches; this Well hath a Cover of Stone.[10]

It is near what was known as the Female Warrior's House. The St Kildans would once point out the stones where she laid her helmet and sword, and it was said that in her time there was a continuous tract of dry land between the islands and Harris where the Warrior loosed her greyhounds while hunting deer.

WHOOPING COUGH

For whooping cough, there were various treatments. The child would be given water to drink in which a toad had been placed. Or the child would be taken across water, all the better if between two parishes or two counties, to a house where it might be offered food, mare's milk, or water from the clefts of a rock – the remedy being the more efficacious if the drink were taken from a horn which had been removed, by accident or force, from a living animal.

Mrs Katherine Whyte Grant told the Caledonian Medical Society in 1904 how not so many years before, a neighbour of hers went through such ceremonies in order to cure her three children of whooping cough:

> She carried each in turn into the middle of the stream, and, having dipped into it a horn shed by her heifer two or three days previously, she made the child drink all the water contained in the horn. She is a Ross-shire woman. She has not the remotest idea that the cure is a superstitious one.[11]

Mrs Grant neglects to say what the outcome of the ritual was but, since she tells it at all and expresses no censure, presumably the children recovered.

11

THE ENCHANTMENT OF
STONE AND METAL

Healing stones and minerals occupy a fascinating position in traditional medicine, linking an ancient veneration for the material itself with the later scientific use of their elements in numerous pills and potions. In the most simplistic sense minerals and plants represent two extremes of creation: the abiding and the transitory, the strong and the fragile.

An Indonesian creation myth delightfully illustrates an elementary understanding of the essential difference. In the beginning, when the sky was very near the earth, God hung his gifts on a cord in order to bestow them on the primordial couple. One day he sent them a stone, but the ancestors, surprised and indignant, refused it. Some days later God let down the cord again, this time with a banana, which was immediately accepted. Then the ancestors heard the creator's voice: 'Since you have chosen the banana, your life shall be like the life of that fruit. If you had chosen the stone, your life would have been like the existence of stone, unchangeable and immortal.'[1]

From scatterings of quartz pebbles in early graves to the great prehistoric megalithic monuments, from tiny microliths through flint arrowheads to jadeite axes, stone has indeed shown how the ancient cultures have made their mark beyond their own times. The perception of those distant societies in terms of Stone, Bronze and Iron and, to a lesser extent, other minerals including pottery, lingers not simply because these enduring items were the mainstay of their technologies but because virtually everything else about them has merged with the earth that supported them. This is especially true of the Highlands, where acid soils make fast work of any organic deposits.

Stones, then, have a magical quality rooted in the earliest conscious-ness of mankind that, while flesh and vegetation were corruptible, the smallest pebble, like the grandest rock, endured. People would not have taken long to perceive that some were more durable, less workable than others, that some, especially when polished, interacted with and reflected the light of the even more magical effects of sun, moon and fire. The raindrop may reflect light as prettily as the diamond, but the latter transcends time.

Mineral objects might be handed down from generation to genera-tion, a tangible link with ever more remote ancestors and virtually untouched by the ravages of time. Sometimes when broken apart they might reveal curious fossilised images that must have seemed truly magical to early peoples.

The gifted Cromarty stonemason Hugh Miller who was to become, among many other things, a fine thinker, essayist, editor, naturalist and palaeontologist, wrote in 1841, of his wonder, twenty years before as an apprentice quarryman in Cromarty, at the inner delights and mysteries of stone:

> In the course of the first day's employment I picked up a nodular mass of blue limestone, and laid it open by a stroke of the hammer. Wonderful to relate, it contained inside a beautifully finished piece of sculpture – one of the volutes apparently, of an Ionic capital; and not the far-famed walnut of the fairy tale, had I broken the shell and found the little dog lying within, could have surprised me more. [2]

He broke open nodule after nodule and found further curiosities. One type of stone, he was told by a fellow worker was 'deemed of sovereign efficacy in curing bewitched cattle'. In the afternoon, it being a half-holiday, he went along the shore and came across thin alternating strata of limestone and 'beds' of a black slaty substance:

The layers into which the beds readily separate are hardly an eighth of an inch in thickness, and yet on every layer there are the impressions of thousands and ten of thousands of the various fossils peculiar to the Lias [Lower Jurassic formations] . . . I was lost in admiration and astonishment, and found my very imagination paralysed by an assemblage of wonders that seemed to out-rival the fantastic and the extravagant even in its wildest conceptions.[3]

Long before Miller people would have learned, as he did, that the black slaty substance in the limestone strata 'burns with a powerful flame and emits a strong bituminous odour'. They learned how to manipulate the soft, incorruptible strength of gold into enchanting forms, to blend copper and tin into bronze and, much later, to form iron into weapons, tools and pots. The metalsmith's art was akin to magic in the minds of lay people, and doubtless the craftsmen played on that awe. In quite early times jet was fashioned into handsome jewellery and the inherent attraction of even common quartz led to mysterious scatterings of it at burial sites. The bigger, grander stones were raised in splendid formations enhanced by their setting in the landscape.

How they learned, in a rudimentary but nonetheless astute way, of the intrinsic medicinal and chemical properties of minerals will probably remain a mystery. But the Gaels were the inheritors of a very ancient wisdom and their medicinal use of the stones and metals in relatively late times, bridges a gap between the early experimenters and the laboratory researchers of our own day. The science and magic of stones is a truly unbroken thread between the most distant past and ourselves. People may have invested certain stones with magical properties in a way that seems mere superstition to us, but their awe of what remains beyond the grasp of the human mind portrays, in the origins of such concepts at least, a proper humility. In unleashing the very authentic powers of materials such as uranium and plutonium, modern science has perhaps gone to the other extreme. So much depends on the language in which convictions are expressed.

The rest of this chapter gives the chief ways in which minerals, in various forms, contributed to the vast materia medica of the Gaels and their predecessors in the north and west of Scotland. Stones are listed first, followed by other minerals and metallic objects. Unlike the contents of most other chapters in this section, the materials are not listed alphabetically.

LARGER HEALING STONES

The Clach-bhan or wife stone, near the Linn of Avon between Braemar and Tomintoul, which was much resorted to by pregnant women in hope of gaining safety and immunity from pain during labour, is typical of many standing stones and natural boulders to which healing properties are attributed throughout the Highlands and islands. Infertility cures were also prominent, presumably because of the phallic symbolism of the stones involved. Sometimes any stone would do. A patient suffering from lack of appetite, failing health, and 'a nervous feeling that all was not well', was advised to go down to the sea shore, take his pants off and go astride a rock or large stone which was half submerged in the shallows. The late Revd Norman Macdonald recounted that '[the patient] had to do this for a short period each day. Apparently such cases were actually improved by this method.'[4]

Stones also appear to have had some kind of importance in the healing of toothache, perhaps because of a loose resemblance, despite difference in size, between tooth and rock. The following charm from Glen Urquhart was, like most of those for toothache, written in English (rarely Gaelic) on a piece of paper to be worn by the sufferer:

> St Peter sat on a marble stone,
> Jesus Christ came to him alone,
> 'Peter, what aileth thee to weep?'

'My Lord and God, it is the toothache.
Rise up, Peter, and not you alone,
But everyone who in this charm doth have belief
Will from the toothache never lack relief.[5]

The 'marble stone' appears an essential part of some of these toothache charms and may be related to the practice of transferring sickness or pain to an inanimate object.

HOLLOWED STONES

Water taken from the clefts or hollows of rocks was believed to be more efficacious than 'ordinary' water in a number of remedies such as whooping cough or wart removal. The same idea applied to hollows in dressed or carved stones like the querns used for grinding corn, baptismal fonts and certain grave-stones. Virtually every home once had its quern which collected rain-water when left outside. Baptismal fonts in ruined, roofless churches, performed the same function with the added quality of a certain sanctity.

Trumpan church in north Skye has an old stone font which is said never to run dry whatever the weather. Coins were dropped in to bring luck and good health, though now this practice is said to be confined to tourists. In the adjoining churchyard there is the Priest's stone which has a small hole into which blindfolded people put their index fingers. If they missed it was said they were sinners, doomed to eternal punishment.

In Islay there is a subtle link between the orthodox medieval medicine and the vestiges of a folk belief that, as likely as not, long preceded as well as outlived the clan physicians. The finely carved Kilchoman cross, of a style that has been dated to the second half of the fourteenth century and standing over eight feet tall, has at its base man-made hollows or cups, one of which has a stone which has to be turned sunwise while making a wish, rather in the manner of working a mortar and pestle. The incomplete Latin inscription on the stone translates: 'This is the cross by Thomas, son of Patrick, doctor, for the souls of his father, mother, wife, and of all the faithful departed, and of the said . . . '

At Bohuntin in Glen Roy, an area with a particularly strong tradition of folk medicine down to the early years of the twentieth century, one can still see the cruisie mould in the blacksmith's anvil used by Domhnall mac Eoghainn Mackintosh from nearby Bohenie. A very small man known as *Luisreagan* (herbalist), he was one of the Kylachie House Macintoshes and lived in the second half of the nineteenth century. Domhnall pounded his herbs in a part of the anvil that served as an iron mould for *crùisgeinean*, iron oil lamps. The anvil, which is said to date back to the time of the battle of Mulroy in 1688, is made of iron, but the principle of its ability to impart some special quality would be the same as that relating to stone. A stone used in Glen Roy for preparing herbs (perhaps by Domhnall mac Eoghainn, among others) has been slightly hollowed by wear. The top of the stone is stained red by continued use for processing plants.

Small pebbles with natural perforations were sometimes chosen as charms and most of them seem to have been worn smooth by water. The stone amulet belonging to Coinneach Odhar, the Brahan Seer, who is believed to have lived in the seventeenth century, was said to have been of this type. Some stories say he would see his visions through the hole in the pebble but in most cases the hole simply seems to have served as a means for threading a cord to hold the charm round the wearer's neck.

VOTIVE OFFERINGS IN STONE

There were stones specially shaped to represent parts of the human body. Such practices were well entrenched in the continental and insular societies of the Celts dating back to at least the Iron Age. Votive offerings of limbs and organs, representing diseased parts of the body, were made at the great healing cult sites of Gaul and Britain, just as they were in the classical Mediterranean ones like the shrine of Asclepius at Epidaurus.

A pair of ivory breasts found at Bath may have been offered by a young mother or a woman suffering from breast cancer. Fontes Sequanae, a Romano-Celtic healing shrine north-west of Dijon dedicated to the goddess of the Seine at the point where the river has its source, has revealed a wealth of models of eyes, breasts, heads, limbs and internal organs carved from wood.[6] These have been preserved by the waters into which they were cast.

In the Gaelic tradition such practices lasted until quite recent times. Late into the last century people still visited Millmore near Killin, in Perthshire, on St Fillan's Day (9 Jan.) to be cured by dark stones which, it was once said, had been sculpted to represent the human head, arms, legs, thumb, heart and so on. The Killin stones were widely believed to have been used for healing since the time of Fillan himself, an eighth-century missionary of the Celtic Church. Later inquiries suggested they were originally 'socket stones in which the spindle of the upper millstone used to work before the introduction of the improved machinery'.[7] The patients washed in a waterfall and whichever stone represented the sick part was rubbed on it while the skin was still wet. One old woman who administered the cure in the nineteenth century would rub the appropriate stone three times *deiseil* (sunwise) and three times *tuathail* (anti-sunwise) round the afflicted area, then the whole body, while reciting charms.

The fact that the healing formalities were carried out in the shade of an ancient elm was deemed a further potent influence. Duncan Macintyre, a nineteenth-century miller who assisted at these rites, is recorded as saying: 'Whether one believed or not in their efficacy to cure, it did no harm to give the stones a clean bed once a year.' However, the miller's casual-seeming remark may be a veiled reference to a parallel and widespread Celtic practice of ritually washing sacred and healing stones once a year. According to Geoffrey of Monmouth, when Merlin advised King Aurelius to remove the 'Giant's Dance' (Stonehenge) from Ireland to Salisbury Plain he said:

> They are mystical stones, and of a medicinal virtue . . . [they] make baths in them, when they should be taken with any illness. For their method was to wash the stones, and put their sick into the water, which infallibly cured them. With the like success they cured wounds also, adding only the application of some herbs. There is not a stone there which has not some healing virtue.[8]

Votive stones did not necessarily have to have a special shape. Many ordinary stones smoothed by sea or river were left as simple offerings on cairns.

On the altar of St Ronan's chapel in the island of Rona, near Lewis, there used to lie a plank of wood some ten feet in length with holes cut at twelve-inch intervals. In each hole was a stone to which various powers were ascribed, one of them being especially valued locally in former times for its claimed ability to grant women in labour a speedy delivery.

In the island of Bernera, south of Barra, a local stone was used for rubbing the breasts as a preventive against disease. It was believed to be so efficacious as a preservative of good health that it was said to be the only medicine in use there when this practice was recorded 300 years ago.

PAINTED PEBBLES and **'COLD-STONES'**

The painted pebbles that have been found at archaeological sites of the first millennium AD are unique to the north of Scotland. Pictish in provenance, they are small rounded quartzite beach pebbles painted with simple but carefully executed designs in a dye of which only a dark brown stain survives. The patterns consist of dots and wavy lines, a pentacle motif, crescents, arcs, triangles and an encircled cross. One is entirely covered with 'crazy-paving' lines.

The archaeologist Anna Ritchie, an expert on the Pictish period, believes that Calum Cille's use of a white stone to cure a Pictish druid (see Chapter 3 above) 'reflects a contemporary climate of thought in Pictland in which the idea of pebbles acquiring special properties was by no means alien. Columba's pebble was not painted, but it does provide a convincing context for the painted pebbles found on archaeological sites.'[9]

Dr Ritchie points out that in Scotland 'cold-stones' – natural pebbles selected for their aesthetic shape and coloration – were used particularly in curing sick animals: 'Water into which such a pebble had been dipped was believed to have healing powers when given to cattle to drink; the pebble acted as an omen as well, for if it dried quickly the animal would recover swiftly, and if it dried slowly the animal would make only a slow recovery.'[10]

A stone of this type, an oval light-brown pebble, about 42 by 63 mm (now in the Museum of Antiquities in Edinburgh), belonged to an Angus farmer in the 1870s. He kept it in a small leather bag around his neck.

In the West Highlands quartz pebbles were put in the drinking water of cattle with red-water fever, and I understand this practice is still sometimes employed. The reasoning behind such cures may not be too fantastical. After all, we have been warned of the trace elements imparted to food and liquids cooked in aluminium pots. The pebbles could well impart some tiny trace of minerals to the water in which they are boiled. Having witnessed someone rally round from sunstroke after being given water to drink in which a quartz pebble had been heated, I am inclined to give the practice the benefit of the doubt, though the liquid alone may have been responsible.

SMALL HEALING STONES and AMULETS

The smaller 'pocket' healing stones were sometimes, like the *Clach Dhearg* (Red Stone) of Ardvorlich (a crystal now in the Museum of Antiquities), mounted in silver, sometimes polished, sometimes plain. Whatever their individuality, they were believed by their owners and the people who resorted to them to be possessed of special powers. A number of families passed charm stones down through countless generations. One of these was the Keppoch stone, said to have been taken to Australia by a branch of the Macdonnells of Keppoch in the mid-nineteenth century. The custom was for this silver-mounted rock-crystal to be dipped in the waters of *Tobar Brighde* (St Brigid's Well) while calling on the 'powerful, beautiful, yellow gem' to heal all the ills of every suffering creature in the water kept pure by Brigid in 'the name of the Holy Apostles, Mary the virgin of virtues, the high Trinity and all the radiant angels'.

Although this well was situated in a part of Lochaber which to this day remains strongly Catholic, a factor which has often helped to keep very ancient traditions alive in the memory in islands such as Barra, Eriskay or South Uist, its exact whereabouts are no longer known despite strenuous efforts to track it down.

Another famous amulet was the *Ball Mo-Luidhe* of Arran, a spherical green stone described by Martin as being 'about the bigness of a Goose-Egg'. Like a number of other amulets, it was credited with a sacred origin, and its virtue, according to Martin, was to remove stitches from the sides of sick people by setting it close to the affected part; 'and if the Patient does not outlive the Distemper, they say the Stone moves out of the Bed of its own accord, and *è contra*'.

The Arran stone was also used for swearing oaths and if it was cast among the front line of an enemy onslaught, it was believed the men would lose all courage and run away. A family of Clan Chattan, otherwise known as Mackintosh, kept the stone on behalf of the Macdonalds of the Isles who were said always to be victorious when they threw it in front of their foes. When Martin visited Arran towards the end of the seventeenth century the *Ball Mo-Luidhe* was in the custody of Margaret Miller, or Mackintosh, who kept the stone wrapped in fine linen with an outer covering of wool and locked in a chest when not required to 'exert its qualities'. Like the Keppoch stone, its whereabouts are now unknown.

There were other famed stones, such as *Clach na Brataich* (the Stone of the Standard) of the Robertsons, and the *Clach Bhuaidh* or Stone of Virtue, a crystal ball belonging to Campbell of Glenlyon (for more about rock crystals see below). 'As a rule,' writes Thomas Davidson in 'Animal Treatment in Eighteenth-Century Scotland', 'where these stones are used as cure amulets, they are either dipped in water, and the water given as a drench to the animals, or the affected part of the animal, or sometimes the whole animal, is rubbed with the stone.'[11] Human patients received much the same treatment and while the cherished stones never went far from their owners, 'guardians' might be a better description, bottles of 'treated' water often travelled some distance to effect a cure.

Tiny flint arrowheads, relics of early hunters, were believed to be fairy arrows, and were considered lucky to have about the house. The Welsh made an ointment for painful joints containing flintstone pounded with primroses and chickweed and while, so far as I know, there are no records of such cures in the purely Gaelic tradition, flint may well have been used in a similar way.

Certain illnesses in cattle were believed to have been caused by 'elf-shot' – the flint arrowheads, often turned up by the plough, which were believed to have been fired at cattle by the fairies.

> The body of a cow so shot at swelled, and the animal would not eat. The shot did not pierce the outer skin. The cure consisted in the finding of the subcutaneous lesion. An intensive search of the cow's body was made with the fingers, and if a spot was found where the finger sunk into a hole in the muscle below the skin that was the elf-shot wound, and the result of finding it was the speedy recovery of the animal.[12]

Pieces of white or rose quartz, known as 'fever' or 'hectic' stones, were put in boiling water to impart a special quality. When the water cooled people washed their arms and legs in it and believed it prevented rheumatism and other ills. At other times the water was drunk – not after washing in it – to help cure a fever. Adomnán relates how Calum Cille healed the Pictish king's druid, Broichan, by dipping a white stone in water from the Ness and blessing it in the name of Christ.

In some places it was known as 'the white stone of the fairies'. The tradition goes that a fairy gave a piece to a herd boy who was amusing himself by pouring water from a neighbouring burn on to a fairy knoll. The fairy appeared at his side and said, 'Thank you, little boy, for the refreshing water you have been pouring on the roof of my house. Here is a stone of great price. Your father has pains in his flanks: let him rub this stone on the seat of pain, and drink of water in which it has been dipped, and he will soon be well again.' The boy took the stone home, it was used as directed, and not only cured his father, but was found to be a panacea for all similar cases in the district. The stone was carefully kept in the family, who refused to part with it on any terms, at least until the end of the nineteenth century when the story was recorded.

ROCK CRYSTAL

Perhaps the most famous of Scotland's many rock crystal charms is the large one surmounting the sceptre of the Scottish Regalia. A close rival is the one on St Fillan's crozier, now in the Museum of Antiquities, but such stones have been found in more ancient and far humbler situations.

A cone-shaped rock crystal was found over a century ago in a Bronze Age crannog (loch-dwelling) in Lochspouts, near Maybole in Ayrshire. Just under an inch in diameter and three-quarters of an inch long, it has a slightly convex base and was deliberately ground to shape. Munro's *Ancient Scottish Lake-Dwellings* records that 'it depolarises a ray of light'. Rock crystal was used as a burning lens for sacrificial purposes according to Orphic literature which also mentions it as an external application for kidney disease, and Pliny recommended a ball of rock crystal held to the rays of the sun as medium for cauterising wounds.[13]

Many crystals were used as protective charms, healing agents and jewellery throughout the Highlands and islands, sometimes combining all three uses. In Gaelic rock-crystal balls were known as *léigheagan*, healing objects. Unlike traditions in England and elsewhere in which crystal balls were valued for supposed fortune-telling properties, the Gaels do not seem to have used them for this purpose, although the brilliant light given by the *Clach na Brataich* of the Robertsons before Bannockburn was said to have foretold that victory. Before the battle of Sheriffmuir in 1715, when the Jacobite army lost to a Hanoverian force, a large internal flaw was observed for the first time and the crystal was never carried to battle again, although it continued to be used as a curing stone. According to a manuscript of between 1749 and 1780:

> They ascribe to this Stone the Virtue of curing Diseases in Men and Beasts, especially Diseases whose causes and symptoms are not easily discover'd; and many of the present Generation in Perthshire would think it very strange to hear the thing disputed.[14]

The stone was carried about by the clan chief or members of his immediate family[15] and is last known to have been used in healing sometime between 1822 and 1830, when the then chief ceremonially dipped it in a huge china bowl full of water from a fairy spring. Afterwards, the water was 'distributed to a number of people who had come great distances to obtain it for medicinal purposes'.[16]

SERPENT STONES and SERPENT BEADS

Few objects have had more nonsense written about them than the so-called serpent-stones and beads but it is rather delightful nonsense. Pliny seems to have started it all. In an account which ends with his saying that the Emperor Claudius put to death a commander of the

Vocontian Gauls for carrying a 'serpent's egg' as a talisman while involved in a legal argument, the Roman writer delves in all seriousness into druidic romancing. In summer numerous snakes entwine and generate the beads from their saliva. According to the druids, Pliny continues, the hissing snakes then cast the beads into the air where they must be caught in a cloak before they touch the ground. The hollow serpent-stones were used by snakes for sloughing their skins. And so on, in the same vein. Such beliefs were still prevalent in the Highlands centuries later. It is now known that the hollow 'adderstanes' are prehistoric spindle-whorls, and the beautifully coloured beads, Iron Age glass ones. It is just possible that snakes emerging from the holes where they have wintered might sometimes dislodge long-buried ancient artefacts, thus giving rise to the legends.

The Gaelic name for serpent-bead is *glaine nathrach*, meaning 'serpent's glass'. The prehistoric spindle whorl is *clach nathrach*, literally serpent-stone. In earlier times no one would have known of the real origin of these artefacts, had they done so we would have been deprived of many ingenious tales. Several of the spindle-whorl stones in the Museum of Antiquities originated in Lewis where they had been used as charms for the cure of snake-bitten cattle – in an island where there are no venomous snakes. Various sicknesses of humans, sheep and cattle in Lewis and other of the Outer Isles were once put down to the bites of non-existent adders, especially where symptoms included some kind of skin peeling or flaking. The custom, as elsewhere, was to put a red woollen thread through the hole, dip the stone in water, bathe the affected part and give the patient some of the water to drink. Similar customs once existed throughout Europe and, needless to say, this is not a belief current in Lewis today.

Hugh Macaskill of Bracadale, Skye, acquired one in about 1859 that had been in his family for years as a cure for 'elf-shot' cattle by dipping it in the beasts' drinking water. Only a year before the then Free Church minister at Bracadale had ordered the people to deliver up all the 'elf-shot', adder beads and charms in their possession as he was determined to 'root out the devil and all his superstitious rites' from among them. One account says he got two creels full, another half a boat-load, which he took to the middle of Loch Dunvegan and dumped overboard.

Snail-stones (*cnaipein seilcheig*, small hollow cylindrical glass beads use for healing sore eyes), cock's 'knee-stones' (*clachan-glùin a' choilich*, small fossils used for sundry disorders), and frog or toad-stones (*clachan nan gilleadha cràigein*), the teeth of fossil fish supposedly used for stemming bleeding and drawing poisons all fall into the same category.

BELLS

Anyone who has ever felt deafened by the clanging of bells will realise their overwhelming effect on the ear. After all, they were designed to attract attention. The ancient medical precept of like curing like that long preceded the theories of modern homoeopathy, meant that what could cause deafness might also heal it. It is possible that a form of cupping with a bell might have helped certain ear conditions. In another Celtic medical tradition, that of Brittany, pilgrims with ear troubles were known to put their deaf ear into a wall cavity at the chapel of St Cado, at Reclus near Auray, to obtain relief.

The bronze bell of Adomnán, kept at Insh church, Kincraig, was believed to have healing powers, as were the bells of Calum Cille and St Patrick, the last being used for expelling demons and also healing rheumatism if passed three times around the body. The *Life of Mochua of Balla* claims:

> Now Taithlech, son of Cennfaelad, suffered from a gangrene, and Mochua healed him, and put the disease on his own bell, and thereon it is still, to certify that great miracle.[17]

BULLETS

Colic was treated by making the patient swallow a bullet, presumably a small one, from the idea that its weight would unravel the knotting of the bowels – believed to be the cause of the colic. It is not hard to see the reasoning behind this and it is just possible that the size, shape and weight of the bullet would indeed have helped to remove certain obstructions on its journey through the guts but it does seem a rather extreme measure. I have not found any record of whether this was actually known to have worked but the fact that it appears to have been accepted as commonplace by a doctor who remarked on it in the late nineteenth century,[18] would suggest that it did, indeed, have a certain reputation for efficacy.

COINS

Certain preparations of water, in which coins of gold, silver and copper had been placed, formed the basis of a cure for the 'evil eye'. (See Chapter 10.)

GOLD

Sore eyes were healed by putting gold rings in the ears, or by rubbing the ears with jewels of pure gold, and repeating certain rhymes. Styes were rubbed with gold rings and the same remedy was applied to ringworm.

IRON

There was a widespread belief that a rusty nail taken from a coffin in a churchyard, and placed under an aching tooth, would relieve the pain. Jaundice was relieved by dashing cold water over the body, or by passing a hot iron over the spine and giving the patient a drink made from a decoction of the common slater in beer.

LEAD

Insanity was formerly believed to be a disease in which 'the person's heart was out of its proper position'. In order to get it back, the following ceremony was performed by some 'wise', i.e. sane, person. Following an invocation to the Trinity, some melted lead was poured into a wooden vessel containing water, which had been placed on the patient's head, and if any of the solidified lead in any way resembled a heart, it was taken and turned round, with the result that 'the patient's heart returned to its place', and the disease was cured. This piece of lead was carefully preserved afterwards, so as to prevent relapses. This example of 'casting the lead' has been taken from the *Journal* of the Caledonian Medical Society and a similar one was recorded at the end of the nineteenth century by the Revd James Macdonald, Reay (on the north coast border of Caithness and Sutherland) as having been used in attempts to heal typhoid fever.[19] A Ross-shire doctor said it was practised on epileptics in that county.

SALTS

Various medicinal salts were kept in the houses of the better off, but common table, cooking or sea salt was significant to the poorer people both in its use and avoidance.

For appendicitis a tablespoon of salt was taken 'out of a bottle' every hour. My informant who remembers hearing of this cure in her younger days thinks the salt may have been suspended in water and was taken to make the patient vomit.

There are several instances of cures or invalid diets where salt was to be avoided. People suffering from the stone or wasting diseases, for example, were not to take salt in their brose.

Angle-berries, a disease of horses which gives them a jerky move-ment, was treated with a daily dose of Epsom salts. When a purgative was needed for humans, Epsom salts dissolved in a decoction of senna leaves was a common remedy in later times.

SALTPETRE

Galar an earbaill, tail fever in cows, is a type of milk fever arising from shortage of minerals after calving. The old cure was to cut the cow's tail above the soft part, rub in saltpetre, or soot and fresh butter, and bandage.

SILVER

In the area around Inverness scrofula was once treated by wearing a silver coin suspended by a silk cord round the neck. A more complex cure involving silver was practised in attempts to heal epilepsy. Finger or toe-nail parings and a new sixpence were carefully wrapped in a piece of paper on which was written, 'In the name of the Father, Son, and Holy Ghost', and placed under the wing of a black cock, which was then taken backwards to the place where the patient had had the first fit. Then the cock was buried alive by the oldest God-fearing man in the district, who had to watch all night by a fire which was not allowed to go out.

12

OF MICE, HORNS AND BUTTERFLIES

The Edinburgh Pharmacopoeia of the late seventeenth and early eighteenth centuries included materials which, had they been found in some poor old woman's house, might readily have led to accusations of witchcraft. For in that book is found, to name but a few curiosities: bodies and eggs of ants, snakes' skins, hooves of elk, spiders' webs, woodlice, horse, goat, pig and even human excreta, powdered Egyptian mummy and extracts from the skulls of those who had died a violent death.[1]

It is against the background of such orthodox medical practice that the Gaelic cures derived from animal materials must be seen, and it must be borne in mind that the modern pharmacopoeia, too, contains animal-derived extracts under the guise of Latin names, white powders and odourless liquids. The common use of spiders in the old Highland medicine might be said to have gained a belated scientific respectability through present-day research in the United States into the therapeutic value of spider-venom in treating strokes and epilepsy. Laboratory-extracted snake serum as an antidote to snakebites may provoke no sense of surprise today, but the former Highland custom of soaking adders' heads in water to provide a remedial potion shows a similarly scientific and deductive line of thinking, however much the old society lacked refined technology.

Listed below are some of the commoner remedies derived from mammals (including humans), birds, insects, reptiles, and fish.

BALLAN

Agnes Maclennan, who now lives in Achmore in Lewis, remembers a variety of old cures that were still being practised in her native Bernera in the 1940s. Once a very widespread procedure, the *ballan*, or cupping with a cattle or sheep horn, is still very occasionally employed in the Outer Isles. Agnes Maclennan recalls:

> You just put a *ballan* on a knee that had fluid or any joint that was thought to have fluid, say the elbow. The one I have heard about is the knee. I saw my old aunt have her knee cupped, using a sheep's horn. The man came to the house, in Bernera, complete with his sheep's horn, knife and methylated spirit. The knee was cleaned with the spirit, he scratched the knee with the knife in the appropriate place, he placed the horn, wide-open end to the knee and through the narrow end of the horn he sucked the fluid out of the knee. It certainly worked for my aunt but I was concerned as to why – was she afraid the horn would come back! Seriously, I do know it worked for many.

Alexander Carmichael tells of the twenty-six year-old Muriel Macleod who was treated by the cow's horn *ballan* of Murdoch Maclean in Breanish, Lewis:

> If I leant forward my eyes filled with water and I could not see, and I had great pain and dizziness in my head. The doctors at Stornoway, Lochs and Tarbert treated me twelve times with the *cuileaga Spàinneach*, fly-blisters, but all to no purpose; if no worse, I was certainly no better. I then went to Murdoch Maclean. He placed the *ballan* on the back of my neck, and sucked through it until he had raised a large lump. He pricked this lump with a needle. Replacing the *ballan*, he again sucked strongly and steadily. He applied the *ballan* in all five times, four times on the first night and once on the following night, this time upon the other side of my neck. He thus drew two saucers full of clear water streaked with blood. I felt severe pain, as though racked from head to foot. The marks of the *ballan* were deep in my flesh and the needle marks lasted a long time, but they were bathed and bandaged until they

healed. I now feel as well and as healthy as I have ever felt in my life, and more than grateful to my kind benefactor Murdoch Maclean.[2]

Sometimes heat was applied to the horn, or a small lighted taper put to the inside to create a vacuum, but most accounts tell of the vacuum being caused by sucking out the air, which would certainly have been less alarming to the patient. The part of the body being treated swelled to fill the vacuum. The *ballan* of Murdoch Maclean of Breanish was a cast cow's horn with an opening drilled at the point, and a piece of *streafon* (the membrane covering the calf at birth, and as tough as it was fine) stretched over the base.

On a more intimate note, the *ballan* was sometimes used by men who found difficulty in achieving an erection. It was a desperate measure, and an island doctor who, some years ago, was called to visit a rather embarrassed patient suffering from an over-energetic application of a *ballan*, would strongly advise against the method.

BEE

Beeswax, hog's lard and locally obtained pine resin were mixed to make a plaster for boils and sores. The plaster was spread on four-inch squares of linen, leaving a margin of about an inch. One of these was then warmed at the fire and applied to the boil, being left in place for twelve hours, when it was removed and burned. The skin area was then bathed and another plaster applied.

A healing ointment was made from docken roots, boiled till soft and mixed with equal parts of beeswax and fresh homemade butter. Honey, both as a sweetener and a nourishing restorative, was included in a number of remedies.

BEETLE

'Spanish fly' preparations made from the cantharides beetle were in use in the Highlands from at least the time of the medieval doctors.

Dr H E Fraser of the Caledonian Medical Society noted that 'fly-blisters' placed on the neck and both wrists were in common usage in the Inverness area in the late nineteenth century.

BIRDS

The young of the solan goose or gannet – a bird which is not strictly speaking a gull, but related to the pelican – is still known in the north west by its Gaelic name of *guga* and to this day remains a culinary delicacy in Lewis. In the old days it provided, with the fulmar, something of a flying medicine chest, especially for the people of remote St Kilda who appear to have used little in the way of herbal remedies.

The St Kildans ate a pudding made of guga fat stuffed into the bird's stomach and boiled in a water-gruel, while the liquid was taken as a medicine for coughs. On its own, the fat was used to heal cuts and wounds. (See also **EGG**.)

Fulmar oil, also burned for lighting, provided an ointment for aches and pains in bones and muscles, and was used for purging and provoking vomiting. In the seventeenth century the oil formed a valuable part of the St Kildan economy, being delivered to London and Edinburgh where it was successfully employed in treating rheumatism, sprains, dental abscesses and boils.

The fat of black-throated divers was valued as a relief for sciatica and even the common crow had its medicinal uses. Its burnt ashes were said to be good for gout.

BLOOD

Some people were believed to have the power of arresting any flux, including severe haemorrhages, by repetition of certain words and the administering of a bowl of the patient's own blood, which had been boiled, dried, and powdered. Swine's blood was supposed to wash warts away. In Lewis the best-reputed cure for shingles was the application of the blood of a black cock, or the blood of a person named Munro, to the affected area. (See also **GOAT** and **HARE**.)

BUTTERFLY

The butterfly exemplified the ideas of shape-shifting and metamorphosis that fascinated the Celts. Other sacred creatures might be killed for food or remedies, not so the butterfly. To kill one was to strike at what the creature represented, although its caterpillar phase (see below) seems to have been less revered.

Fearchar Lighiche was said to have been transformed into a blue butterfly after his death. Many souls – and angels – were said to take the form of butterflies, the colour of the wings denoting the character of the individual (e.g. white for good, dark for bad), and the colour blue was often associated with healing.

There are numerous Gaelic words for a butterfly but some of the most common are, *dearbadan-Dé* (God's butterfly?), *amadan-Dé* (God's fool), *anaman-Dé* (God's little soul), dealan-Dé (God's lightning or – electricity) and *dealbhan-Dé* (God's little image). Children had a rhyme they would recite while circling a burning stick in front of a fire; the original Gaelic wording varied from place to place but might be roughly translated as:

> Butterfly, butterfly,
> My blessing to the Son of God,
> My blessing to the house of God,
> And my blessing to you.

You might chase the very words for butterflies – *dealan* and *dealbhan*, *amadan* and *anaman* – around in the head until they become as elusive as the creatures themselves. Then, again like the butterflies, they alight and are caught in a sense of wonder. The connections of meanings and the intrinsic dance and colour of language touch on something that seems akin to healing itself.

Dwelly's *Gaelic-English Dictionary* (1901–11) gives *dealan-dé* as 'the appearance produced by shaking a burning stick to and fro, or by whirling it round', which reminds one of children delighting at the patterns made by twirling sparklers.

The butterfly has a place in this list not because it was ever used in any way as a physical remedy, but because its imagery encapsulates the essential riddle of what medicine still calls the *vis medicatrix naturae* – the healing force of nature.

CATERPILLAR

A belief in the power of a caterpillar wrapped in a small piece of red cloth, or of a rusty nail taken from a coffin in a churchyard, and placed under the offending tooth was once widespread.

CATTLE

Milk held an important place in the Gaelic materia medica and was used both internally and externally as a treatment for a variety of problems. The cow was deemed such a 'blessed' animal that it was forbidden to slap it by hand. This taboo was got round by tapping the beast with a stick.

Persistent coughs were treated by a drink of warm cow's milk in the morning, or a concoction of two parts milk and one of water, mixed with a little treacle and vinegar, and drunk warm. 'Consumptions, and all disorders of the liver, found a simple remedy in drinking of buttermilk,' wrote Thomas Pennant in 1772.

In early times a bath in milk was highly regarded. The *Chronicon Scotorum* records that, following a battle in which poisoned arrows had accounted for a number of casualties, a Pictish druid directed a large hole to be filled with the milk of 150 white-faced cows. The wounded were bathed in it and said to be cured. On another occasion an Irish warrior, Cathan, was immersed in a bath of cow's marrow and cured of his wounds. Cream was boiled until oily, then cooled and applied to burns.

A strip torn from the breast of a cow killed at Christmas was singed and sniffed by everyone in the household as a security against evil spirits. Alexander Forbes says in *Gaelic Names of Birds, Beasts, etc*, that a spoon made from a horn lost by a living cow was thought to heal many diseases when food was eaten from it. When the cow died the efficacy of the horn spoon ceased.

It was said of cattle: *Uilleadh na bà a-mach 's a-steach, mur leighis sin an Gaidheal chan eil a leigheas ann.* (The oil of the cow within and without, if that won't heal the Gael, there's no cure for him.) For the uses of butter, see under **FAT** below.

A belief in the healing power of bulls is discussed in Chapter 6. The milk of pure white cows was particularly valued, and it is interesting that Robert Sibbald, writing in 1684, records in his *Scotia Illustrata* that wild white herds of cattle roamed the hills. Stories of these animals may have given rise to the 'fairy cattle' of legend.

CAUL

The caul, or membrane which sometimes covers the head of a newly-born infant, was greatly prized by the Gaels and particularly by seafarers. It once had a considerable market value owing to the belief that it offered a certain protection against drowning. The caul of a child was of special value, but those of animals were also treasured. Dr S. Rutherford MacPhail recalled in 1896 that he had seen a caul tied up to the rafters of a Highland hut.[3] In the 1970s a woman on the east coast of Sutherland was known to carry her own caul about in a special purse which she always kept in her handbag.

People 'born with the caul' were believed to have certain healing powers. In the case of Neil Mòr, an Eigg man who died as recently as the early 1960s, the fact that he was 'born with the caul' only added to the status of having been born of a long line of hereditary healers. The family were noted for curing bad backs by walking on them. My informant remarked, 'Neil, by virtue of his weight, some eighteen stone, probably did not have many clients . . . '

CHICKEN

Many manifestations of diseases of the nervous system were often attributed to the working of evil spirits, and epilepsy, being an alarmingly sudden and generally striking disease, was looked on as ripe for propitiation or exorcism. A once common practice was for a black cock to be taken reverently to the place where the person had suffered the first 'attack', whereupon the bird would be killed and carefully buried, a series of prayers and incantations being repeated during the ceremony.

This notion of an 'attack' derives from the once widely spread belief that certain diseases, but especially epilepsy, were quite literally due to an assault by a malignant spirit. We still talk of an 'attack' of asthma, a heart 'attack' and, indeed, an 'attack' of epilepsy. The practice of medicine has moved on, but both its lay and professional language remains imbued with some ancient beliefs. Even the word 'epilepsy' itself comes from two Greek words meaning to be 'seized upon'.

At Dunbeath Market in November 1851, a crowd gathered round a man suffering an epileptic fit and made numerous suggestions as to what should be done. Some of the older witnesses insisted on the traditional custom of getting a black cock with no speck of white about him, digging a hole in the spot where the man fell, and burying the cock alive in it. This was actually done in the presence of hundreds of people. The underlying theory was that the malady was transferred to the cock and buried with him.

Bruises and injuries were healed by applying fat extracted from the inside of a hen. One cure for a snakebite was to kill a fowl, split the warm carcass, and immediately place it over the wound, keeping it in position while it gradually drew out the poison. People with stomach ulcers, and 'bad' stomachs, were fed chicken meat and broth. Rather as in the Jewish tradition, mother's chicken soup was considered of great benefit to a number of conditions.

Chicken and chicken stock were highly esteemed for people who were terminally ill, being easy on the digestive system. When there were cockerels available at times of illness, they were sent live to the patient's house and killed as necessary.

CORPSE

Drinking from a suicide's skull was a treatment common to many localities, and varied on the West Coast by giving the patient water to drink in which a corpse has been washed. The practice was usually carried out as a remedy for epilepsy. Scrofula victims were believed to benefit from touching the hand of a dead criminal.

DEER

For sprains, a thread on which three knots had been tied, in the name of the Trinity, was fixed round the limb above the affected joint, but the method was believed to be most efficacious if the thread were a sinew from a rutting stag. Deer tallow was often used for healing chilblains and protecting the skin against the ravages of weather.

Stag-horn jelly was a nourishing and widespread part of the invalid diet. It was made by smashing a quantity of newly cast antlers with a hammer, putting them into a large pot and covering with water. After boiling for about three hours, the liquid was strained into a basin before being put into a pot with candied sugar and a little vinegar. It was brought to the boil again and then allowed to set in a basin till it formed a thick jelly. The remedy was administered a tumblerful at a time. This was taken to the boil and given with the addition of some whisky. It was especially good for any chest troubles including tuberculosis. In a slight variation of a proverb applied to cows, it was said: – *Geir féidh a-muigh 's a-staigh, mur leighis sin thu chan eil do leigheas ann.* (Deer fat [applied] outside and inside, if that doesn't cure you, there's no cure for you.)

DOG

Dogs have peculiar links with healing that stretch back into ancient history. Asclepius was said as an infant to have been suckled alternately by a bitch and a she-goat, and his images were often accompanied by a dog. Is there, perhaps, any connection with the modern medical advice to keep a companionable dog as a therapeutic aid for a nervous or stressed disposition? Several old legends involving a divine or human protagonist with healing attributes mention the stealing of dogs. Just as Hercules stole Cerberus, the watchdog of Hades, so Brian, Iuchar and Iucharba – grandsons of Oghma, the insular counterpart of the Romano-Celtic Ogmios, whose link with healing seemingly lay mainly in his influence over magical words and incantations – were sent to steal the hound-whelp of the king of Ioruaidh.

A faith in the curative power of dog's saliva – perhaps a magical 'inversion' of the knowledge that a rabid dog's saliva is fatal – may have lain behind Celtic beliefs in the healing attributes of the animals. Rabies was alleged to be cured by placing a 'blessed' cloven stick on the tail of the infected animal, which stick bore the somewhat singular term of *seangan* (thin one or ant). So many and wondrous were the old cures for rabies that doubtless a number of them gained their reputation from the fact that the patients they 'cured' had been bitten not by a rabid animal but simply a rather cross one.

EGG

The following cure from Shawbost, Lewis, was told to me by a man now living in another part of the island:

I remember as a very young boy in the late 1930s or early 1940s having a very bad bout of diarrhoea for a few days. Then I used to do messages, and take in the water for my aged grandparents, and when I told my granny the problem that I had, she just said 'wait a few minutes'. Then, she put an egg in a pan, and after a while she made me eat the hardest boiled egg one could eat – and that was the end of my problem. My grandmother's cure for my discomfort was one of the things that happened to me in my young days that I shall never forget. It was instantaneous.

Another informant, from Bernera, said the egg would probably have been boiled in milk which would have been drunk alongside the eating of the egg.

In St Kilda, raw gannet eggs were considered a great cure for chest infections.

EXCRETA

Archaeologists investigating native sites contemporaneous with neighbouring Roman ones in the south of Scotland have remarked on the lack of Celtic artefacts in rubbish and votive pits compared with those of the invaders. One conclusion is that the Celts threw away very little, leaning heavily on recycling any likely material in a waste-not want-not society. The Gaels worked on the same principles, though the fact that their medical preparations included excreta, both animal and human, does not make them unique. Such materials were widely used in ancient healing traditions and, much as it may surprise more delicate modern minds, they may not have been without some value.

Fresh cow-dung was supposed to be particularly soothing for an inflamed breast. Scabs or blotches on the face were cured by applying cow's dung in the summer season. One reason given for the seasonal use was that in summer the dung has healing power from the great variety of medicinal herbs eaten by cattle. Similarly 'May' butter was considered the best as it was made from the milk given by the cows who grazed on the early summer herbs.

Quinsy – suppurative tonsillitis or an abscess in that area of the throat – was, it was claimed, usefully treated with a poultice of cow's dung applied externally to the throat. 'Foul shave', a condition which my informant (a woman) thinks may refer to boils on the neck or face caused by careless shaving, was also cured with an application of cow's dung. The white in hen's dirt was used for drawing pus.

A cure for blindness, once practised in the west Highlands, was to dry and powder human excrement and blow it in the eyes of the afflicted person. 'They were very poor people. They had nothing, nothing, and they tried anything,' was the explanation from an informant. This may have been true of such practices in the troubled years of the nineteenth century *Gaidhealtachd* but, *pace* early pharmacopoeia, was based on theories once held in orthodox medicine.

Lightfoot's *Flora Scotica* records that 'a poultice of human ordure is a sovereign remedy for the bite [of a snake]'.

Ernest Marwick's excellent book, *The Folklore of Orkney and Shetland*, devotes a chapter to traditional remedies in the Northern Isles in which he remarks:

> . . . until the early part of the last century (in a few places much later than that), some people continued to believe in the medicinal value of excreta. A bleeding nose was plugged with fresh pig dung, a bruise was poulticed with cow dung . . . and milk in which sheep droppings had been boiled was drunk by people suffering from smallpox.[4]

FAT

Various fats were used as a base for healing ointments. Perhaps because the wild deer has little fat, its grease was the most highly valued. Bruises might be treated with a slice of bacon, or a good thick layer of salt butter, either of which helped to keep down the swelling. Fluxes were sometimes treated with a poultice of flour and suet, or newly churned butter, or strong cream and fresh suet boiled together, and applied plentifully morning and evening.

The *deoch dhubh*, 'black drink', may owe as much to its alcoholic as its fat content. Recipes varied, this one is from Inverness-shire:

> Put homemade butter in a pan and take to the boil, then skim and put the pure oil in another dish, keeping the grounds out. Clean the pan and put in it clean oil, a whisky glassful, and add the same amount of whisky. Take both to the boil and drink as hot as possible first thing in the morning on an empty stomach.

Soap and sugar, or butter and oatmeal, were good for drawing pus. Hacks on hands or feet were soothed with deer tallow, or resin used for sewing leather, or, again, an oatmeal and butter poultice.

A very old cure for all venomous bites, but especially those from adders, was butter churned on a Friday from the milk of a one-coloured cow (a white one for preference). No water was allowed in the churning and a special incantation was sung over it nine times.

FISH and SHELLFISH

The juice of the cuddy, or saithe, was taken for indigestion. In *Folksongs and Folklore of South Uist*, Margaret Fay Shaw says that *greim-maothain*, a pain suffered by spinners through swallowing bits of wool while holding it between their teeth, was cured by eating boiled cuddies, bones and all. (In the chapter on herbal cures mention is made of the confusion that can be caused by local variations on plant names. Here is a 'fishy' version: in many parts of Scotland 'cuddy' is the name given to the donkey, while in most Gaelic-speaking areas it is the saithe or coalfish, from the Gaelic word *cudag*.)

Dogfish oil was given to people with asthma. The juice of boiled herring was drunk as a remedy for stomach disorders and salt herring was taken for bile. The Revd Norman Macdonald, a native of Skye, said that the fat of a conger eel was very much used for bruises and other injuries 'with excellent results'. A South Uist man told me, 'For a sprained ankle, an eel was caught and skinned. The eel skin was put round the ankle and as it dried it became tighter. It was left there till it rotted and fell away. Eel oil was also used for arthritis.' There was an intriguing cure for tuberculosis recalled by the Revd Norman Macdonald: 'Along with a conger eel, there was boiled the patient's semmit or undershirt. The semmit was taken straight from the pot and worn all the time, day and night. I have heard of a man who was perfectly healed in this manner.'

Limpets were put to heat on a cinder, then the oil was dripped into the ear to help dissolve wax. These shellfish were an important part of the economy and diet; as well as being used for line-baiting, they made a nourishing broth. Martin wrote:

> The Limpet being parboil'd with a very little quantity of Water, the Broth is drank [sic] to increase Milk in Nurses, and likewise when the Milk proves astringent to the Infants. The Broth of the black Periwinkle is used in the same cases . . . I had an Account of a poor Woman, who was a Native of the Isle of Jura, and by the Troubles in King Charles the First's Reign was almost reduc'd to a starving Condition; so that she lost her Milk quite, by which her Infant had nothing proper for its Sustenance: upon this she boil'd some of the tender Fat of the Limpets, and gave it to her Infant, to whom it became so agreeable, that it had no other Food for several Months together; and yet there was not a Child in Jura, or any of the adjacent Isles, wholsomer than this poor Infant, which was expos'd to so great a Strait.[5]

FROG

For dropsy a frog was cut in half and a piece placed on each side of the patient's belly. A cure for red water fever in a cow was to thrust a large yellow frog down the beast's throat. This practice was witnessed by a vet when he was a student in Argyll in the 1940s. When asked whether it worked, he said: 'I don't know. The frog kept jumping back out of the cow's mouth and I left the men when they were looking for the frog in the hay for the umpteenth time!

The skins of certain frogs and toads are known to contain several substances, such as bufotene, which have been and are being employed in pharmacy, so the use of frogs may have had a sound basis if somewhat curious methods of application.

In a variation on the Highland practice of using the tongue to lick a foreign body from someone's eye, it was claimed that it worked all the better if the eye of a frog was licked first.

The ashes of a burned frog were, it is said, sometimes used to stem severe bleeding but, given the numerous herbal and other applications for this purpose it is unlikely that this cruel method was resorted to with any frequency. Frogspawn was one of many remedies for erysipelas and other inflammatory skin conditions.

Many years ago a group of local men working in a desolate stretch of land in north Sutherland sent the youngest of their company off to fetch a kettle of water to make tea. They all praised his skill at tea-making and asked for more. Off he went again to collect water, and what should he find when he took the lid off the kettle? A well-boiled frog at its bottom. Saying nothing of his discovery to his workmates, he extracted the frog, refilled the kettle and made more tea. No one was any the worse of it, except – the second mug of tea was not so highly praised.

GOAT

Goat's milk was taken as a tonic following influenza but was also credited with wider healing values: *Is leigheas air gach tinn cneamh agus im a' Mhàigh; agus òl am fochair siud 'm bainne ghobhar bàn.* (A cure for every patient is garlic and May butter; and drink along with that the milk of white goats.) The blood of wild goats was supposed to disperse kidney, bladder and gall stones. Herds of goats were still kept for their milk in the Highlands and islands at least till the end of the eighteenth century, and during the summer invalids would make journeys to drink the 'medicinal' milk.

HARE

Hares were sacred animals to the Celts. In earlier times they appear to have been more strongly connected with hunting and military symbolism but later they became closely associated with the supposed shape-shifting abilities of poor and elderly women healers. It was believed that a 'witch' who had turned herself into a hare could be harmed only by being shot with a silver bullet.

The use of the hare in medicine was common to the Arabian and Celtic traditions. The gall was used to treat eye-problems, the blood to treat skin blemishes and the brains for severe headaches. Urine retention and kidney or bladder stones were remedied with a mixture of the hare's blood and skin.

This advice for the treatment of vertigo or migraine is one of the prescriptions of the Welsh Physicians of Myddfai:

> Take a live hare, behead it, skin and boil or roast, then open the head, taking some rosemary flowers, and powder the same, put them in the head, mixing with the brain, and baking or roasting it. Let the brain be then eaten, the patient sleeping afterwards, and it will be found really useful.[6]

HORN

Water, taken from the clefts of rocks specially to treat whooping cough, was said to be more efficacious if drunk out of a horn which had been removed, by accident or force, from a living animal.

HORSE

Horses and their riders held a special place in Celtic healing lore. The Celtic Apollo, a sun-god and healer who went by various names, was often depicted on a horse and an ancient folk-memory may lie behind the later tradition, which survived into the nineteenth century, that a stranger on a piebald horse had the power of curing whooping cough by advising the correct remedy.

> Fhir tha marcachd an eich bhric
> Ciod as leigheas air an t-srut-chasd?'
> (Rider of the piebald horse,
> What is a cure for whooping-cough?)

A similar custom comes from Corgarff, Aberdeenshire. A person with a sore eye or stye would say to a man riding a white horse: 'Man, man, wi' the fite horse, tak' styan aff my ee.'

Mare's milk was deemed the best drink for someone severely beset by the spasms of whooping cough. There is at least one instance of a sickly infant being, it was said, successfully reared on mare's milk, his own mother being unable to nurse.

LEECH

As well as being usefully employed in the therapeutic bleeding of patients, leeches were made into a broth (by boiling the creatures in water and straining off the liquid for drinking) which had a good reputation as a cure for tuberculosis and other wasting diseases and was also given for persistently bad coughs.

MOLE

Rheumatism was treated by applying earth from a molehill, as hot as could be borne, to the affected part, then poulticing with seaweed.

MOULD

Long before the discovery of penicillin, people kept saucers of milk until it grew a mould. In the Calgary area of Mull this mould was applied as a poultice on ulcerated legs. The various moulds growing on the walls of caves were believed to be excellent for wounds, and 'cave soil' was said to be particularly effective for damage to the limbs.

MOUSE

Boiled, fried or roasted mice were a specific for whooping cough from Shetland southwestwards across the Highland mainland and out to the Western Isles. In some places mice were also given for jaundice and smallpox. In December 1922, Donald A Mackenzie gave a lecture entitled 'Oriental Elements in Scottish Mythology' to the Gaelic Society of Inverness, in which he compared a practice he had seen as a small boy in Cromarty with archaeological discoveries at the pre-dynastic (c.4000 BC) Egyptian site at Naqada.

What he saw as a child was a woman cutting the liver from a mouse to give to a neighbour's baby who was believed to be on the point of death. The baby, recalled Mackenzie, recovered and grew to be a healthy boy. Many years later he was to read with deep interest of the discovery of the ancient cemetery in Egypt where a number of adults and children had naturally mummified in the sand. Professor Elliot Smith, who dissected and analysed the bodies, reported '. . . the occasional presence of the remains of mice in the alimentary canals of the children, under circumstances which prove that the small rodent had been eaten after being skinned.'[7] Smith then added a remark that fascinated Mackenzie, 'Dr Netolitzky informed me that the mouse was the last resort of medical practitioners in the East several millennia later, as a remedy for children *in extremis.*'

In the old days, Highland children did not leave a milk tooth under the pillow for the tooth fairy, but placed it at a mouse's hole asking the wee creature to take the small tooth of a happy child and give a big strong one in return. In *The Golden Bough*, J.G. Frazer gives similar examples from as far afield as Germany and Raratonga, in the Pacific. In the former country a child was to throw its fallen milk tooth backwards over its head behind a stove, saying: 'Mouse, give me your iron tooth; and I will give you my bone tooth'. In Raratonga, the child would beseech: 'Big rat! little rat! Here is my old tooth. Pray give me a new one.'[8]

OTTER

Otters were once believed to have a magic skin which acted as a charm against death by drowning or troubles in childbirth. The skin was also used to make a potion for fevers and smallpox. Anyone who licked the warm liver of a newly killed otter was said to gain the power of healing burns and scalds by licking them three times. In Eriskay, Father Allan MacDonald recorded:

> I saw a man with a trifling scorch on his finger go in jest to two men who had gone through the otter ceremony, and they seriously enough licked the finger. This is an old belief by no means extinct. Today [26 Feb. 1896] I saw the ceremony of licking the finger done, and the men were surprised I had never heard of it before.[9]

PIG

Pigs were believed to cause ills as well as cure them. A bite from the animal was once said to induce cancer. On the other hand, an application of its blood was supposed to remove warts. Many legends about pigs may originate in their prehistoric status as a tribal totem. The Pig or Boar tribe would have had a taboo on swine-flesh except as a ceremonial dish at special feasts. One of the tasks of the Children of Tuirenn in the legend that has been called the 'Gaelic Argonauts' was to fetch a magical pigskin renowned for curing all ills and having the rather agreeable knack of turning water into wine. Another task was to acquire the seven pigs of Easal, King of the Golden Pillars, which might be killed every night yet found alive and well again next day. (The antics of the cartoon characters, Tom and Jerry, seem to echo the Celtic otherworld of Tìr nan Òg where slaughter and fighting always resulted in the physical renewal of the combatants however severe or fatal their injuries.) Anyone who ate a part of the seven pigs could never again be afflicted with any disease.

SALIVA and SPITTING

A person suffering from toothache was advised to make an oatmeal bannock mixed with saliva and place it in water under a bridge where the living and dead cross – all in silence. As the bannock melted and disappeared, so too, it was hoped, would the toothache.

Inflammations of the eye were 'benefited' by a 'person who had the power' spitting and sprinkling soot on a stone which was then rubbed on the affected eye first thing in the morning.

SEAL

The dried and pulverised liver of a seal was drunk in milk or whisky to remedy fluxes. Whatever the efficacy of that, there is no doubting that swallowing seal oil was found to be an excellent preventive and even, it was claimed, cure for colds. Externally, the oil was rubbed on chests for bronchial colds, used as an embrocation for sore joints, and as a soothing agent for burns once the skin had cooled.

SHEEP

Long before official medicine treated the condition known as myxoedema (a thyroid deficiency) with thyroid derivatives, the people of, at least, Uist and Kintyre, treated the disease they called *brisgein* with the thyroid gland of a sheep. This is one of the most outstanding examples of the astute and advanced medical thinking of the Highlands that was hampered only by lack of scientific technology.

Scraps of fleece caught on heather, shrubs and dykes were collected for tying round hard and obstinate corns. Lamb broth in which lovage had been boiled was given to people suffering from tuberculosis, and said to be very effective nourishment.

A tale frequently heard in Skye in former times was of people who imagined they had swallowed a tadpole when they went down on all fours and drank without a dish from wells and streams. The tadpole was then believed to develop as a frog inside their bellies. The remedy was as follows: a black sheep was slaughtered and a joint of it roasted; a piece of the roasted meat was then placed on a plate, given to the patient who held it directly below the mouth, when all of a sudden the frog on smelling the roast, jumped out.

Strange as it may seem this appears to have been based on an old cure for appetite problems which embraced both anorexia (a phobia of food) and bulimia (binge-eating followed by induced vomiting). In the older form of the cure, meat was roasted but *not* immediately given to the patient. In this way it was hoped to excite a renewal of appetite and interest in a balanced diet, and the patient would only be allowed to eat once it was established that a cure had been effected.

In his *Popular Tales of the West Highlands*, John Francis Campbell recounts a story connected with Fearchar Lighiche who had been called to see a daughter of Mackay of Kilmahumaig, near Crinan. Fearchar's servant remarked, as they approached the house, on the sound of a woman singing:

> "'S binn an guth cinn sin,' ars an gille.
> "'S binn,' ars an t-Ollamh, 'air uachdar losgainn.'
> ('Sweet is that head's voice,' said the lad.
> 'Sweet,' said the doctor, 'above a toad.')

Campbell continues:

The poor young woman had an enormous appetite, which could not be satisfied, but she was reduced to a skeleton. The doctor, on hearing her voice, knew what her disease was, and ordered a sheep to be killed and roasted. The lady was prevented from getting any food, from which she was in great agony. She was made to sit by the sheep while it was being roasted, and the flavour of the meat tempted the toad she had swallowed to come up her throat and out of her mouth, when she was completely cured. The reptile she had swallowed was called *lon craois*.

Lon chraois is both a term for various aquatic creatures ('water-spider, water-beetle, water-demon, water-glutton') and for morbid gluttony and bulimia. The symbolism of the frog may stem as much from early attempts at graphic description of a sensation, as from simple fancy or superstition. We still call hoarseness 'a frog in the throat'. In a couple of hundred years time – perhaps less, given the rate at which idiom is changing – they might think us rather strange for that.

SKULL

Drinking from a suicide's skull was a treatment for epilepsy in many localities. It was varied on the west coast by giving the patient water to drink in which a corpse had been washed. In Kirkwall, in Orkney, part of a human skull was taken from the churchyard, grated and administered to the epileptic. In terms of modern transplant surgery such cures do not, however crude in their form, seem so bizarre in concept. Water from the skull of a suicide was also given to the insane. The reasoning behind this may have stemmed from a belief that the mental and emotional state of a suicide, or anyone who had died a violent death, may in some way have altered the chemical make-up – as it was understood – of the 'vessel' used. In former times cups made from different woods were believed to impart the 'virtue' of that wood to its contents.

SLATER or WOODLOUSE

Jaundice was relieved by dashing cold water over the body, or by passing a hot iron over the spine. Internally a decoction of the common slater or woodlouse, in beer preferably, was given. Slaters were also sometimes given in cases of whooping cough. Quite what its value was believed to be is hard to say. Perhaps it was assumed to work in the same way as the spider (see below).

SNAIL or SLUG

In many parts the slug and the black snail are known by the same Gaelic name, *seilcheag*, and medicinally they were often used in the same way. They are both still being used successfully in some areas for curing warts and even corns. A woman in Castlebay, Barra, and a young boy in Kinlochbervie, west Sutherland, both had warts cured by slugs or snails in the past few years, and they are only two of many people in the Highlands and islands who set great faith by a method which appears to have none of the magical connotations of most so-called wart cures. (See under LILY in Chapter 14 for an old corn-cure involving black snails.)

Long ago snails were roasted by a fire and the juices that dripped from them were given to people suffering from lung diseases. At one time, it is said, all the Celtic peoples made a nourishing soup from snails but now, only the French – who inhabit what was once Celtic Gaul – seem to consider them a delicacy. Dr H.E. Fraser, of the Caledonian Medical Society, commented: 'Nourishing foods and fat substances were found to be of great value [in treating tuberculosis]. The oily drippings of snails chopped up fine and hung in a flannel bag in front of a fire, and [bone] marrow, being the forerunners of the now ubiquitous cod-liver oil.'[10]

The oil or juice from snails was also considered a valuable embrocation for chronic rheumatism. A more curious use was to apply bruised snails to the legs to remedy whooping cough. In Uist jaundice was treated by giving patients drink from water into which large shelled snails had been put while still alive.

External swellings and tumours, and especially tubercular tumours on the back, were poulticed with a number of split black snails. A bandage was placed over the snails to keep them in place and fresh applications were made as often as necessary until the swelling healed. In Orkney and Shetland snails in vinegar were administered for rickets. In Uist cold sores were cured by rubbing with a slug.

SNAKE

Adders' heads were preserved for years to heal adder bites. If a person or any domestic animal was bitten, the dried snake's head was steeped in water, then the liquid drained off and the wound washed in it. This method had a great reputation for healing and may somehow have worked as a crude forerunner of the modern antidote using extracted serum. In principle, at least, the old idea anticipated one of the discoveries of modern medicine. Neil Matheson, writing in the Scots Magazine in 1949, said:

> The writer recently met several people in the district of Kilmuir, in Skye, who distinctly remembered the *pocan cheann* – the bag of heads – as it was called and had seen it used on many occasions. The bag contained the heads of an adder, a toad and an esk (or newt). When cows or humans, were suffering from wounds inflicted by any of these creatures the *pocan* was dipped in a stream at a place where it divided two crofts. The water which escaped from the bag when it was lifted out of the stream was then applied to the wound.[11]

Several herbal cures for snakebite will be found in Chapter 14. A very much more prosaic method, which doubtless gave some relief in the case of minor bites, was simply to apply baking soda to the wound.

One rather suspect Highland cure was the belief that if the bitten person could reach the nearest water, a burn or pool, say, before the snake did, and wash the wound, he or she would be healed immediately. Given that the last thing a snakebite victim should do is move about quickly – thus hastening the spread of the venom through the bloodstream – this is a curious piece of advice from a medical tradition that owed much to common sense. However, folk memory may owe something to a druidic belief that, according to Pliny, when a thief fled on horseback, serpents could pursue him only as far as a river.

An ointment made of serpent grease was supposed to give the power of seeing the supernatural. It is possible that some kind of mind alteration could have been induced, as occurs by using the skin of some toads and frogs which contain an hallucinogenic known as bufotene. (Serpent stones and beads are dealt with in Chapter 11.)

SPIDER

A spider encased in a well-sealed goose-quill and hung round a child's neck was reckoned a certain cure for the thrush. It might be argued that a mother prepared to go to such lengths would, in any case, be a caring woman, and thrush will clear up all the more readily if the child is generally well looked after.

Modern investigations into spider-venom extracts, including the north American common garden variety, have proved their value in the treatment of stroke and other neurological problems. During a stroke, brain cells degenerate and die around the damaged area due to shock and lack of oxygen. The damage is worsened by the body's own over-production of natural glutamates, which, released at a toxic level, overstimulate and further destroy cells. Spider-venom seems to be the answer, since in the last few years it has been discovered to contain properties which, when injected into the nervous system, act as glutamate blockers.

In the old days one cure with a great reputation among the Gaels for helping whooping cough, was to swallow a live spider. Perhaps the venom released by the understandably panicking spider soothed the coughing spasms. The difference in method between modern and traditional medicine may be wide, but the theories behind the practices developed from comparable intellects. Indeed, the old healers may be accorded higher honours since they lacked academic libraries, and microscopes and other mechanical aids to research.

Cobwebs – fresh, not dusty old ones – were placed over a cut to stop bleeding and, by all accounts (including recent incidents recounted to me), this worked very efficiently. In some places people used cotton threads drawn from cloth for the same purpose.

TOAD

A live toad was held before the face of someone with a nosebleed – perhaps the idea was to stop the bleeding by startling the patient as in the well-known method of putting, say, a cold key, or poker, down the back. Giving a child drinking water in which a toad had been put was one way of trying to relieve whooping cough. Maybe something in the toad's skin helped to allay spasms.

URINE

Katherine Whyte Grant recalled a case where a boil had refused to come to a head or succumb, after two attempts, to the doctor's lancet:

> An old neighbour happened to call on the mother whose child was suffering. She advised her to make an oatmeal poultice with urine, instead of water, and promised it would bring speedy relief. The mother, without delay, applied the remedy. It quickly softened and cleansed the boil, and there was no more trouble about it.[12]

Rheumatism was treated with a hot mixture of stale urine and bran applied to the painful part. Chilblains were relieved by putting the feet in a chamber pot of hot urine, or washing soda and hot water, every night until they eased. Deer tallow was then applied as protection from further trouble. In the Northern Isles sweetened urine was a remedy for jaundice.

Urine, which in any case is some 96 per cent water, contains valuable minerals of which the most important is urea, a substance in daily use in modern medicine for a variety of treatments. This is now made up from a chemical formula but modern pharmacy cannot ignore its base in the astute experiments of folk medicine. Today, urea remains an important ingredient in medicinal skin creams and treatments for ulcers and infected wounds.

I can remember babies having their faces wiped with their own wet nappies in the belief that this practice would give them good complexions. A friend of mine with four boys made a virtual religion of daubing their faces with their damp nappies and not one of those boys became a spotty teenager. The nappies would have to be recently wet since urea is quickly changed by a yeast-like micro-organism into carbonate of ammonia, the substance that gives off the distinctive bad smell.

WORM
Boiled worms were a remedy for stomach disorders. A stranger who claimed to be a seventh son of a seventh son was tested by an earthworm put in the palm of his hand. If the man was telling the truth, it was believed the worm would die at once.

13

RITUALS, CHARMS AND INCANTATIONS

The importance of words, numbers and movements at the very centre of the Gaelic healing tradition indicates a culture where science and the arts were at one – where numbers were magical and words were chosen with precision. To us in the late twentieth century, this 'centre' is imbued with glamour and mystery, as indeed it was probably always intended to be. However, when these rituals and chants were still very much a real part of the old medicine, they were also a convention, part of a protocol. All of this had a twin-edged legacy. It contained the seeds of decline so far as practice was concerned, and it engrained the forms deeply in the memory.

Where the Highland empiric experimented widely and shrewdly with herbs and other materials, the old magical-realism of the essential philosophy of the medicine, however we might sentimentalise its holistic nature, allowed for little if any progress. Where art, religion and science, to use the terms broadly, were so closely bonded, there were few incentives for each to prove its superiority over the others. As the old society disintegrated and its learned orders, the respected keepers of tradition, moved away or lost their status, so a number of the old practices, viewed first by outsiders as mere superstition, became to be so regarded by the people themselves – at least in public. The growing influence of the Presbyterian church and southern-influenced education as well as a stream of other cultural influences from the second half of the eighteenth century onwards did not, however, lead to a total lack of confidence in the old ways. The incantations were passed on to those who could be trusted and muttered hastily over the heads of those who were desperate for help.

The following examples rely heavily on the verses collected by William Mackenzie, the first secretary to the Crofters' Commission after it was formed in 1886.[1]

Beguiling as they are, Carmichael's translations and, it has to be said, 'improvements', tell us as much of the pastoral and spiritual yearnings of his own times as they do, splendidly enough, of past beliefs and a poetic approach to life. Mackenzie's slighter collection and his more straightforward English renditions seem more clearly to echo the mind of the past.

For reasons of space, few of the Gaelic originals are given here, but there is some redemption in the sense that their English presentation can make one even more conscious of the fact that the Gaelic versions collected in the late nineteenth century were themselves a relatively recent expression of formulae that would have stretched back to the time of the druids and, quite likely, beyond. If the *Carmina Gadelica* transports the reader to a Celtic otherworld where the natural and the spiritual dance together in a 'green harmony', Mackenzie's collection has us at the mouth of a dark cave from which an ancient voice and the very rocks themselves echo the essential magic of words.

Lucan and other Roman writers tell of the druids' use of hymns, divination and charms for diseases. By the time the incantations came to be written down in the vernacular they had largely undergone a change from a pagan to a Christian context. The names invoked are not, with rare exceptions, those of ancient gods and spirits, but of Jesus Christ and the saints of the early church. As with the metamorphosis of the goddess Brigid into the saint Brigid, so, it would seem, with the pagan elements in the charms. But if the new names were an acknowledgement of changing times, their power was unchanged. To dismiss the use of incantations as mere superstition is to deny the intrinsic potency of language to calm and reassure as much as to disturb and activate.

Popular belief in malignant powers was strong, as shown in this paragraph from a leaflet entitled *Crofters and Witchcraft* which was circulated in Inverness in the winter of 1891–2:

> As an example of how this man of sin punishes those who differ from him in religion, I may state that I am daily tortured by his most powerful agent, viz, witchcraft. It takes away the faculties of my brains; it makes my body feel as if someone was sticking hot irons in me, at other times I feel as cold as ice; it weakens me to such an extent that I am hardly able to move out of the position in which I stand; it gives me such a shock while I am walking on a public road that I am not able to stand and speak to anyone; it has got such a hold upon my body and soul that I find that the most experienced members of the medical profession 'are unable to do any good to me.[2]

Whatever the true cause of the poor, demented writer's condition (he claimed, not surprisingly, to be confined in an asylum), his description is a graphic, if extreme, example of the 'cause and effect' superstitions relating to witchcraft. By such means, certain unscrupulous people gained influence or revenge. Fortunately for the victims, benign rituals were more prevalent, and the Evil Eye curses could be counteracted by any one of a wealth of 'antidote' charms.

The following was sung as a bottle of water was filled and the performer modulated his or her voice 'so as to chime with the gurgling of the liquid as it poured into the vessel':

> Let me perform for you a charm for the evil eye,
> From the breast of the holy St Patrick,
> Against swelling of neck and stoppage of bowels,
> Against nine *conair* and nine *Connachair*,[3]
> And nine slender fairies,
> Against an old bachelor's eye and an old wife's eye.

If a man's eye may it flame like resin,
If a woman's eye may she want her breast,
A cold plunge and coldness to her blood,
And to her stock, to her men,
To her cattle and her sheep.[4]

Vindictiveness or envy, the latter being believed to be the source of the Evil Eye, were not, however, always repaid in like sentiments. The following incantation is typical of the more positive and quite common sort which were not vengeful in tone:

Eye will see you,
Tongue will speak of you;
Heart will think of you —
The Three are protecting you —
The Father, Son and Holy Ghost.
[name of sufferer inserted here]
His will be done. Amen.[5]

It might be said that, more than any other aspect of tradition, the incantations reveal the historical Gaels as fully rounded people. There are charms for the jealous and the lovelorn, the hopeful and the despairing, the caring and the vengeful, the heart and the soul, and the teeth and the bowels. The undoubted psychological value of many charms was often combined with commonsense cures and medicines. Others may simply have had a hypnotic effect or given the patient confidence. Strength of belief alone can be a powerful thing, but an understanding of hypnosis by the old healers would have played an equally important part in certain cures.

William Mackenzie classified the numerous surviving charms and incantations into five types: divination, the achieving of aims, protection, healing and blessings. Among healing charms there were ones for swellings of the breast, in which the affliction was invariably transferred to some nearby, preferably pap-like, hill; charms for eliminating rheumatism, consumption and jaundice; charms against bruising, sprains and dislocations; charms for staunching blood and charms for relieving indigestion. Mackenzie gives examples of each of these and many more. The words were accompanied either by the taking of medicine or the performance of some ritual which could be as simple as making the sign of the cross or yawning, or as complex as entwining coloured threads in a certain way or getting particular kinds of water on particular days of the week, dipping charm stones in water, or using urine, salt or soot in a certain way.

Very little maleficent material has survived but this would reflect shyness of revealing something considered private or even shameful, rather than the lack of a Gaelic urge to curse and condemn. Going by Dwelly's *Dictionary* which lists, though does not give examples of, types of maledictions, there were plenty enough. Under *or* and *ora*, he gives the names of a death spell, a charm to silence an opponent, a wounding incantation, a spell to spoil another's brewing, the 'Friday spell', and a spell to raise a storm or drown a foe.

Healing incantations sometimes display a curious blend of poetic or religious heights and the lowliness of physical functions. In one a 'stoppage of bowels' occurs in the line following 'the love of holy St Peter'. And the charms could be medically detailed. The following is an *èolas* against an ectopic pregnancy – in which the foetus develops in the fallopian tube instead of the womb – in this instance in cows:

Eòlas na Dàire

Eolas na daire 'rinn Moire 's a Mac.
'S thubhairt Criosda fhein gum bu ro-cheart,
Air a'Chiad Luan
'Chur à chruidh gu luath a dhair,
Gun fharlaogh 'n a dheigh
Ach laoigh bhreaca bhoirionn uile gu léir.
(The Charm for the rutting made by Mary and her Son.
Jesus himself said it was right
On the first Monday [or: at the beginning of the moon?]

> To send the cattle quickly to the bull;
> And that no extra-uterine conception should follow,
> But spotted female calves.)[6]

Some of the earliest surviving Gaelic charms still reveal a pagan as well as a Christian influence, giving an intriguing hint of the Gaelic medicine of the druids. The following examples were written in Gaelic in the margins of Latin texts by Celtic monks at the monastery of St Gall in Switzerland. The exact meaning of some of the words is not clear. The first of the four is against a thorn, and as well as Christ it invokes the pagan smith-god Gobniu who formed one of a triad of Irish craft-deities. The humour and exaggeration involved was intentional and typical of the genre:

> Nothing is higher than heaven, nothing is deeper than the sea.By the holy words that Christ spoke from his cross, remove from me the thorn, a thorn which has torn a bloody path (?) . . . a blow there. Go to it, go there, expel it. Very fierce is Gobniu's science, let Gobniu's goad go out before Gobniu's goad!' – This charm is laid in butter which does not melt into water and some of it is smeared all round the thorn without it going on the point or on the wound, and if the thorn is not there one of the two teeth in the front of his head will fall out.[7]

The second is against strangury:

> 'I ward myself from this disease of the urine; wood, cattle (?) ward us, birds, birdflocks, cunning sorcerers ward us.' – This is always put in the place where you urinate.[8]

The next is against headache, a very bad headache by the sound of it. The words of the charm were to be recited in Latin:

> 'Head of Christ, eye of Isaiah, forehead of Elijah, nose of Noah, lip of Job, tongue of Solomon, neck of Matthew, mind of Benjamin, breast of Paul, grace of John, faith of Abraham, blood of Abel: holy, holy,

holy, Lord God of Sabaoth.' – This is sung every day about your head against headache. After singing it spit into your palm and put it round your two temples and the back of your head while singing your paternoster three times, and make a cross with your spittle on the crown of your head, and then make this sign, $\cup$, on your head.[9]

The last is purely pagan in influence:

I save those who are sick unto death from flatulence, from spear-thong, from sudden tumour, from wounds caused by iron, from ul(?) which fire burns, from egg(?) which dog eats; be it the blood(?) that wanes, three nuts that crack(?), three sinews that weave(?), I strike its disease, I vanquish bloods, weeping of bloods. Let it not be a chronic tumour. May what it goes upon be healed. I put my trust in the remedy which Diancecht left with his people in order that whatever it goes upon may be healed.' – This is always put in your palm full of water when washing, and you put it in your mouth, and you put the two fingers next to your little finger into your mouth, apart from each other.[10]

In some instances written rather than spoken charms were believed to be more efficacious, and they were usually sealed before being handed over to the person seeking their benefit. Very often they consisted in a passage from the gospels and it was not unknown for Protestants to request them from baffled Catholic priests in the lingering belief that if they were written on spare leaves from missals they would be more effective. Such protective charms or phylacteries were also common in Greek and Hebrew traditions, favourite quotations being from Exodus xiii: 2–10 and 11–17, or Deuteronomy vi: 9 and 16.

The Jewish practice was to wear phylacteries on the left arm or, when praying, on the forehead. The Gaels, too, wore the written charms about their persons. The charm had to be written by someone else, and if the subsequent owner opened it and read the words the protective or healing power was said to be lost. Toothache charms, such as the one quoted in Chapter 11, were often used in this way.

Incantations were frequently used in connection with bonesetting, massage and manipulation, skills for which Highland practitioners were particularly noted. This was one of the more commonly used verses for the purpose:

> Dh'éirich Calum Cille moch,
> Fhuair e cnàmhan a chuid each
> Cas mu seach;
> Chuir e cnàimh ri cnàimh,
> Feòil ri feòil,
> Féithean ri féithean,
> Seiche ri seiche,
> Smuais ri smuais;
> A Chrìost, mar leighis thu siud,
> Gun leighis thu seo.[11]
> Calum Cille rose early,
> He found his horse's bones
> Leg crosswise;
> He set bone to bone,
> Flesh to flesh
> Sinews to sinews,
> Hide to hide,
> Marrow to marrow;
> O Christ, as you healed that
> May you heal this.

There were several slight variations on this. It is highly likely that its derivation is very old and that the original influence was pagan. An almost identical charm found in a tenth-century German manuscript has Phol (possibly a connection with the Greek centaur Pholus) and Woden performing the same tissue-bonding on Balder's horse.

In the *Lacnunga*, one of the Anglo-Saxon leechbooks, there is a worm charm of which the first three words are Irish:

> Gonomil, orgomil, marbumil.

In modern Irish, suggests Patrick Logan in *Making the Cure*, this would probably be: *Goin an míol, airg an míol, marbhaigh an míol* (Wound the worm, harass the worm, kill the worm). Logan remarks that one might speculate how this charm became part of Anglo-Saxon magic. 'Perhaps', he says, 'some of the Irish monks had a reputation as a medicine man, and in any case it is an example of the survival of a forgotten language.'[12] It would be interesting to go even further and inquire how much the 'occult' or 'mumbo-jumbo' content of other English charms owes to the Celtic languages not only of the missionaries but also of pre-Anglo-Saxon southern Britain. It is often forgotten that the 'English' people, too, have a claim to a distant Celtic ancestry, just as many Scots might (and do) profess Pictish as well as Gaelic antecedents.

Charms in an unknown language – sometimes presumed by the unlettered, and probably intentionally, to be 'magical' words – were in certain instances believed to be more effective. This definitely related to toothache charms in the Highlands, almost all of which were written in English. Erysipelas was believed to be all the better for the recitation of a line in Latin.

Those who had the *eòlas* (knowledge of healing incantations) were as generous as those who gave of their practical learning. A woman known as Sandy Skipper's wife, who lived in Latheronwheel, Caithness, in the middle of the nineteenth century, was typical of her kind. She was believed to have exceptional healing powers and her speciality was children's ailments. She used only incantations and mystic rites and, while there is no record of what these were, they can be assumed to be similar to those already discussed. The Revd George Sutherland said of her that 'her services were willingly and cheerfully rendered without money and without price to all who sought them. The belief that she was benefiting her fellow human beings was her sufficient reward'.[13]

One of her incantations would have been the widespread *eòlas an t-snàithein*, or charm of the thread. While three threads, of red, white and black or, sometimes, blue, were entwined about the affected part, the Gaelic incantation was muttered over the patient three times. In English it translates:

> An eye will see you
> Tongue will speak of you,
> Heart will think of you,
> The Man of Heaven blesses you.
> The Father, Son and Holy Ghost.
> Four caused your hurt –
> Man and wife,
> Young man and maiden.
> Who is to frustrate that?
> The three persons of the most Holy Trinity,
> The Father, Son and Holy Ghost.
> I call the Virgin Mary and St Brigid to witness
> That if your hurt was caused by man,
> Through ill-will,
> Or the evil eye,
> Or a wicked heart,
> That you [name] may be whole,
> While I entwine this about you.
> *In nomine Patris,* . . . [14]

In one of the islands[15] the cure of the threads is still practised and the local doctor says there remains a strong faith in it among a number of the people. Known as *bàrr a' chinn*, 'the top of the head', it involves the winding of red threads around the neck while reciting a charm to 'drive the evil spirits' through the top of the head. Such practices serve to show how ancient beliefs linger on not simply by way of a nod in the direction of tradition, but by way of giving a certain measure of comfort. In all but one of the instances I have learnt of, I have been asked not to divulge where they took place.

Again about twenty years ago, an Inverness newspaper photographer casually and good-humouredly challenged an elderly Kiltarlity woman, who was noted for her knowledge of old medicines, to do something about his sciatica. She took him on and wound threads about his thigh while muttering her charm. Not only was he surprised at himself for submitting to the ritual but, as he later assured me, the pain did indeed go completely. But the threads did not last for long. As time went on, they became increasingly worn and loose and fell away. When they did so, the sciatic pains returned. What are we to make of that?

14

HERBAL

This brief herbal lists only plants and their uses known, from oral or written sources, to have been employed in the traditional medicines of the Gaels or their Celtic ancestors. In some cases the uses of individual plants may differ from, say, southern Scottish and English practices. The herbs most highly valued for their healing powers are marked with an asterisk*.

Much work remains to be done in organising a comprehensive 'Highland Herbal'. As already mentioned, most of the medieval Gaelic medical manuscripts, including those which describe the materia medica, still await scholarly scrutiny; and, so far as the traditional healing is concerned, constant confusions arise from misunderstandings over variations in district names of plants. A Gaelic Linnaeus would be more than welcome.

To give an example, *lus nan laogh* is given in Dwelly's *Gaelic-English Dictionary* as (1) golden saxifrage, and (2) orpine; and in Maclennan's *Pronouncing and Etymological Dictionary of the Gaelic Language* (1925) simply as golden saxifrage. A number of other sources also give orpine. Yet in Lewis and Sutherland, and no doubt some other places, *lus nan laogh* is applied only to the bogbean, one of the Gaels' most important medicinal herbs. A Lewis Gaelic-speaker writing to me (in English) of a well-known island tonic, remarked on the '*lus nan laogh* – golden saxifrage' being collected for it. As it happened, I already knew – from various oral and published sources – that the chief ingredient of this drink is actually bogbean. I asked her why she thought the plant was golden saxifrage. 'I looked up *lus nan laogh* in the dictionary,' she said.

Before it is too late – and in Gaelic as in English, fewer and fewer country people are conversant with the names of many formerly well-known plants – I would make a plea for ecologists, botanists and Celtic scholars to join forces and funding to research thoroughly and publish a Gaelic Flora.

The first entry below is given as an example not so much of confusion between different plants, as of the need to clarify the etymology of and define the most accurate modern term for each individual plant.

AGRIMONY (G. *mur-druidheann, muir-droighinn, mùr-dhroigheann, a' gheurag bhileach*; L. *Agrimonia eupatoria*)
This plant was used to some extent in the Gaelic folk tradition by way of an infusion of the dried leaves for 'open obstructions of the liver', and it was included in the extensive and sometimes exotic pharmacopoeia of the medieval Highland physicians – being used, for example, in the treatment of liver problems and as an ingredient in compounds for 'correcting imbalances in various humours'. I have taken a certain liberty in the third of its Gaelic names (above), since Cameron's *Gaelic Names of Plants* gives *mur-druidheann*, with an accompanying and somewhat fanciful – interpretation as 'sorrow of the druids' and Dwelly gives *muir-dhroighinn*, which would seem to translate 'sea-bramble', as well as *mur-dhroighinn*. Since agrimony is a plant known to thrive best in the shelter of hedges and walls, *mùr* seems the most acceptable Gaelic description. *Droigheann* is more of a problem since it stands for 'thorn' or 'bramble' and agrimony is certainly neither of these. However, its seeds are of a prickly, clinging burr-type and it is possible that here *droighinn* describes the 'thorny' burr.

Maclennan's *Dictionary* gives something quite different: *a' gheurag bhileach*. This term, literally 'the sharp-pointed or bitter-tasting-leafed one' is the most accurate either way you look at it – agrimony has sharply serrated leaves and they taste bitter. Agrimony is predominantly a southern plant in the British Isles, becoming increasingly rare the further north of Hadrian's Wall one goes. This would not have been a problem in medieval times when it formed part of the official pharmacopoeia, since many alien plants were either imported or grown in special herb gardens. (Later folk healers tended to rely on easily acquired local plants about which they were extremely knowledgeable, often, out of need, finding uses for them which were unknown elsewhere.) Its links with medicine and magic can be traced to Mithridates Eupator (hence *A. eupatoria*), a king of ancient Bithynia and Pontus (Anatolia), who was a skilled herbalist and said to use agrimony as an antidote to poisons.

ALDER (G. *fearn*; L. *Alnus glutinosa*)
The leaves were used fresh or in poultices to relieve feet 'tired and irritated by walking'.

ALEXANDERS (G. *lus nan gràn dubh* [plant of the black grains/seeds]; L. *Smyrnium olusatrum*)
Alexanders and lovage in a lamb broth were, says Martin, 'found by Experience to be good against Consumptions'.

*ALL-HEAL (G. *Dubhan ceann-còsach* [spongy-headed kidney] , *Dubhan Pceann-dubh* ; L. *Prunella vulgaris*)
There was great faith in this plant for removing all obstructions of the liver, spleen and kidneys. 'Green' wounds were treated with an ointment made of golden rod, all-heal and fresh butter.

ALOES (G. *aloe*; L. *Aloe ferox*)
The bitter aloe, sulphur, senna, and mineral salts were among the medicines the better-off kept in stock in the nineteenth century. Aloes were employed regularly in the official medieval medicine but little used in the native tradition.

*APPLE (G. *ubhal*; L. *Malus sylvestris* [crab], *M. domestica*)
A decoction of apples and rowan, sweetened with brown sugar, was used to cure whooping cough. The *Regimen Sanitatis* of the Beatons recommended cleaning the teeth with apple skins and taking a roasted apple before bed to help sleep and before heavy meals to help digestion. A cure which combines common sense with the psychological value of mystery is found in Malcolm Beaton of Pennycross's manuscript where the writer advises:

> write this on an apple divided into three. On the first piece, Jesus Christus on leo on filius. On the second, on ovis on aries. On the third, on pater on glan on vermeis. Then eat the pieces and it will help a fever.[1]

*ASH (G. *craobh uinnsinn, nuin*; L. *Fraxinus excelsior*)
In many parts of the Highlands at the birth of a child, the midwife would put the end of a green stick of ash into the fire, and, while it burned, catch in a spoon the sap or juice which comes out at the other end. This spoonful was administered to the new-born babe as its first taste of nourishment.

Burnt ash bark was administered for toothache. Ash leaves were sometimes applied as a poultice to snakebites as serpents were said to have a special horror of the leaves of this magical tree. An old Gaelic proverb runs: *Théid an nathair troimhn teine dhearg mun téid i troimh dhuilleach an uinnsinn.* (The snake will go through the red blazing fire rather than through the leaves of the ash.)

BARBERRY (G. *barbrag*; L. *Berberis vulgaris*)
An infusion of the inner bark was taken for indigestion accompanied by bilious vomiting, known as the 'boil'.

*BARLEY (G. *eòrna*; L. *Hordeum distichon*)
Large quantities of boiled barley (bere) juice were recommended to be drunk for kidney disease. In seventeenth-century Skye a mixture of barley meal and white of egg was applied as a first-aid measure for broken bones. Splints were then tied on and kept in place for several days. When they were removed, an ointment of germander speedwell (which is the *Betonica Pauli* mentioned by Martin Martin, see under **BETONY** and **GERMANDER SPEEDWELL** below), St John's wort and golden rod, chopped and bruised in sheep's grease or fresh butter, was spread on a cloth and applied to the injury where it was kept for a few days.

Martin gives an example of a cure used in Harris for drawing 'worms' out of the flesh. A servant 'having his Cheek swell'd, and there being no Physician near, he asked his Master's Advice: he knew nothing proper for him, but however bid him apply a Plaister of warm Barley-Dough to the place affected. This assuaged the Swelling, and drew out of the Flesh a little Worm, about half an inch in length, and about the bigness of a Goose-quill, having a pointed Head, and many little Feet on each side: this Worm they call Fillan [under *fìolan* Dwelly's *Dictionary* gives 'fly, worm, insect, animal, parasite, and bot-fly], and it hath been found in the Head and Neck of several Persons that I have seen in the Ile of Skie.'[2]

*BETONY (G. *lus Beathaig*; L. *Stachys officinalis / Betonica officinalis*)
A medicinal herb known, according to Pliny, to the ancient Celts
who made great use of it as a nerve tonic – and a cure and preventive
for drunkenness and hangovers. It was said to be especially useful for
treating headaches – whether or not caused by over-indulgence in
alcohol. Its leaves were sometimes eaten as a salad and a tea was made
of it for everyday use. Since it grows best in woodlands in limestone
areas which are rare in the Highlands, its widespread use in Gaelic
medicine suggests that it was specially cultivated in herb gardens.[3]

The ointment of 'crushed St John's wort, betony and golden rod
mixed in butter and grease applied to wounds', referred to by many
commentators, originates from a remedy quoted by Martin Martin.
However, the 'Betonica Pauli' he mentions was the term used in his
day for the germander speedwell (q.v., and see also under BARLEY).[4]

BISTORT (G. *glùineach an uisge, glùineag dhearg, luibh an uisge*; L.
Polygonum amphibium, P. bistorta)
This small reddish flower that trails among corn and potatoes was used
for urinary complaints, with, it is claimed, good results. It was among
the pot-herbs advised by the Beaton physicians for a summer diet.

BLACKTHORN (G. *preas nan airneag*; L. *Prunus spinosa*)
The flowers were used as a laxative, and later in the year the berries
were used for fevers.

*BLAEBERRY (G. *braoileag*; L. *Vaccinium myrtillus*)
The berries, which have an astringent quality, were used for treating
diarrhoea and few herbal medicines were believed to be more effective
for a variety of complaints. John Lightfoot says in his *Flora Scotica*

(1777) 'The berries have an astringent quality. In Arran and the Western Isles they are given in diarrhaeas and dysenteries with good effect. The Highlanders frequently eat them in milk, which is cooling and agreeable food, and sometimes they make them into tarts and jellies, which last they mix with whisky to give it relish to give to a stranger.'[5] Blaeberry jelly was given to people suffering from fluxes and the Revd Angus MacFarlane, who contributed a paper on plant lore to the *Transactions of the Gaelic Society of Inverness* in 1924, says an infusion was used for soothing pain.[6]

In the Reay Country Gaelic of north-west Sutherland, the blaeberry is known as *fiagag*, and was once highly rated in that area for dissolving kidney stones. In the islands blaeberry tea was once a common drink, a custom worth reviving for its health value.

*BOGBEAN (G. *lus nan laogh, trìbhileach, pònair chapaill, mìlsean monaidh*; L. *Menyanthes trifoliata*)
One of the most highly valued plants, a tonic made from bogbean is still used in parts of the Western Isles. Barbara Fairweather gives a recipe that was in use in Glencoe village within living memory: 'The plant was put in a stone jar and simmered on the old range. The resulting water was drunk as a spring tonic. Sometimes the stems were boiled for two hours, pulped, left to cool, the liquid strained and bottled for winter. A teaspoon three times a day for a persistent cough was most effective.'[7]

In Lewis the ribbed side of the leaf was said to be good for drawing out pus, and the smooth side for healing. In Badenoch where the plant, known in that district's Gaelic as the *Luibh Mhòr* ('big herb'), was the most highly prized medicinal herb, the root was used as a stomachic bitter and tonic in all cases of convalescence and debility. A homemade beer was in use in which bogbean took the place of hops, and was stored away to be used when required. A fresh infusion, about four ounces of dried root to an imperial pint of water, was the most popular form, and of this a wineglassful was taken generally before meals.

There was a great faith in the bogbean as a remedy for all manner of stomach pains, particularly those caused by ulcers. The root was chopped and simmered in water and the strained liquid was drunk. A similar decoction was given to strengthen weak stomachs. The juice of the roots was also taken for tuberculosis. For boils and skin eruptions, especially those on the back of the neck once suffered by fishermen as a result of friction from nets, creels and ropes, a poultice of bogbean leaves was applied to the sore and the juice was drunk to clear the blood. A pain in the side following jaundice was treated with a mixture of boiled wild raspberry, wild mint and bogbean. In Uist bogbean was taken for constipation. Animals who had a blockage through over-eating were also fed bogbean. In addition to all the foregoing uses, Lewis people say it is good for asthma and heart problems as it 'helps to open up the tubes'.

*BOG VIOLET or **BUTTERWORT** (G. *mòthan*; L. *Pinguicula vulgaris*)
The dust of bog-violet in a golden amulet had 'a potency against which the wiles of evil were vain'. Whoever wore it was deemed to be secure: 'from all despite; from the sorrow of love ungiven; from a foeman's stroke; from the gnaw of hunger; or from drowning, the doom of the sea.' It was used in love-charms, in 'bewitching' cattle, and also in protecting cattle from 'witches'. Its most practical use derived from its rennet-like action on milk.

BOG MYRTLE (G. *rideag*; L. *Myrica gale*)
Credited with the power of keeping away mischievous fairies, it was once used as a substitute for hops in flavouring beer and is also said to

have some effect in keeping summer insects at bay. It was probably more effective as a domestic 'strewing herb' on floors, helping to deter household pests, bugs and fleas. In Islay and Jura it was used as a garnish for food and for storing with linen as a means of driving away moths and finely scenting the cloth. In many areas an infusion of the leaves was used for worming children.

*BONDUC BEAN (G. *Cnò Mhoire, Crosphuing*; L. *Guilandina bonduc*) These and other seeds and nuts from the West Indies and Central America are washed to the western Hebridean shores courtesy of the Gulf stream. The nuts vary in colour, chiefly brown or white, and the most prized had the form of a cross indented on the side. Worn around the neck, they were believed to attract the special protection of the Virgin Mary. The possessor was saved from various calamities, and notably from sudden death. They were believed to be specially useful in the case of women in labour, and the belief in its efficacy in such cases was still practised in Uist early this century. The mother took the nut in her right hand, and repeated the Hail Mary three times. The midwife then took the amulet and made the sign of the cross with it on the sick woman, while at the same time reciting one of several incantations. An infusion in milk was given for diarrhoea and dysentery, especially in children. It is likely that several species of similar nuts may have attracted the one Gaelic name of *Cnò Mhoire* or *Crosphuing*.

BORAGE (G. *borrach*; L. *Borago officinalis*) The Latin *borago* is probably derived from the Celtic root *borso-s*, meaning 'proud'. The Early Irish was *borr*, also meaning proud or swaggering. There was an old saying: *Ego Borago, gaudia semper ago* ('I Borage, always bring joy/courage'). Alistair Maclean, a native of

Mull and father of the thriller writer of the same name, wrote of its use in the Hebrides: '. . . and borage was the courage-giver. Out of it they brew one of the four great cordials. Whoever drank it drew his sword and thought ten men no match for him.'[8]

BRAMBLE (G. *dreas*; L. Rubus fructicosus)
Infusions of bramble root and pennyroyal were given for bronchitis and asthma. Erysipelas was treated with a poultice made from the leaves.

BROOM (G. *bealaidh*; L. *Sarothamnus scoparius*)
Several sources, including members of the Caledonian Medical Society, testify to the success of a decoction of broom as a remedy for dropsy. This treatment was widely used throughout the Highlands. A bunch of broom wrapped round the neck was said to stem nosebleeds. Two drachms of the flowers or seeds were administered to induce strong vomiting.

BUTTERBUR (G. *gallan mòr*; L. *Petasites albus)*
Used in cases of fever and dropsy.

CAMOMILE (G. *camobhil, camobhaidh*; L. *Anthemis nobilis*)
This gentle herb was highly effective for those with sluggish livers or poor digestion. The Revd Angus MacFarlane remarks 'I remember as a boy seeing a packet procured from a herbalist in the south by a relative. He little knew that it grew as a common weed in the fields at home.'[9] 'Stitches', or cramps, were rubbed with an ointment made of camomile and fresh butter.

*CARROT, wild & cultivated (G. *curran*; L. *Daucus carota*)

Poultices being a popular form of remedy in Highlands for internal as well as external ills and muscle pains, numerous different substances were used. The wild carrot was one of the most highly rated, especially for cancerous sores.

Pennant noted in 1772: 'Formerly the wild carrot boiled, at present the garden carrot, proved a relief in cancerous, or ulcerous cases. Even the faculty admit the salutary effect of the carrot-poultice in sweetening the intolerable foetor of the cancer, a property till lately neglected or unknown. How reasonable would it be therefore, to make trial of these other remedies, founded in all probability, on rational observation and judicious attention to nature!'[10]

In Harris, and doubtless elsewhere, the seeds of the wild carrot were a substitute for hops in brewing, and were said to give the ale a 'good relish'.

The carrot generally was held in great esteem. The Michaelmas feast (29 Sept.) was a great annual celebration in North Uist with both men and women taking part in bareback horse-races along the sands. At the end of the day the men would present women with knives and purses, and the women would give the men pairs of multi-coloured garters and bunches of wild carrots.

*CELANDINE, Lesser (G. *searraiche* or *lus an torranain*; L. *Ranunculus ficaria*)

The shape of this plant's tubers suggested fleshy nodules to people in the Middle Ages and so the lesser celandine was used to treat growths on the ears and neck, small lumps in the breast, and piles. The juice was applied externally to the part affected. But this had to be done carefully as, on healthy skin, it would cause sores and blisters. In the case of swellings in the breast the celandine roots were usually placed under the arms.

*CENTAURY (G. *ceud-bhileach*; L. *Centaurium erythraea*)
Infusions were given for stomach and digestive problems, also as a general tonic and aperitif. It had a specific use in promoting appetite in tubercular patients. In Uist a tonic was made from a tincture of pink centaury in whisky and pronounced 'excellent'.

*CHICKWEED (G. *fliodh*; L. *Stellaria media*)
This plant that we look upon as a nuisance was once highly valued for a number of medicinal uses but especially as a poultice for abscesses and sore or inflamed breasts. The traditional way of preparing it was to bruise the plants between a flat and a round stone which were kept scrupulously clean and dust-free for the purpose. As an added measure of hygiene the stones were heated in a fire before use. The mash was put in a wooden dish and inverted on to the breast, the dish or luggie keeping the poultice in place. The water in which chickweed was boiled was drunk as a slimming aid. The plant chopped and simmered in lard made a good healing ointment.

An unusual Inner Hebridean cure to help someone sleep after a bout of fever was to wash the feet, knees and ankles of the patient in warm water to which a large quantity of chickweed had been added. Afterwards, some of the plant was applied warm to the neck and shoulders and the patient was put to bed. Chickweed tea was taken for insomnia.

CHILDREN'S 'SWEETS AND CANDY'
Long before commercially made sweets and candy were available, Highland children had something far healthier to chew in roots and tubers like those of the wild liquorice (G. *carrachan*, see VETCH, tuberous), earth nut (G. *braonan*), silverweed or white tansy (G. *brisgean*), often found in certain ploughed lands in spring. The hard

'bulb' of certain thistles was cut, placed on a flat stone and broken open by pounding on it with another stone. The inside was sweet and good to chew. The leaves of the common sorrel (G. *puinneagan*) were also eaten.

COLTSFOOT (G. *cluas liath*; L. *Tussilago farfara*)

The dried leaves were smoked in clay pipes to relieve asthma, and the fresh leaves, juice or syrup were all taken for a dry cough. Barbara Fairweather, who has collected a great deal of the local history and folklore of the Glencoe area, notes in her useful booklet *Highland Plant Lore* that the dried leaves were considered 'best for rheums'.

COMFREY (G. *meacan dubh*; L. *Symphytum tuberosum*)

A mucilage of comfrey root was applied to broken bones to help them mend.

CORN, in general (G. *gràn*)

The main cereals grown in the area have been barley, oats and rye. Barley is the longest-established crop, since the oats which were to become the valuable mainstay of the Scottish diet were not cultivated here until Roman times. In Lewis it was said that corn grown in previously untilled land would, among other ills, cause headaches and vomiting in those who ate the bread or drank the ale made from it. See under separate species for medicinal uses.

CORNEL, Dwarf (G. *lus a' chraois* [gluttony plant]; L. *Cornus succisa*)

As its Gaelic name suggests, it was believed to be a powerful appetiser.

COWSLIP (G. *mùisean*; L. *Primula vera*)
Writing in 1924, Angus MacFarlane says that though botanists claim the cowslip is unknown in the Highlands, he had found it to grow abundantly in north Sutherland. The Caithness and Sutherland office of Scottish Natural Heritage has confirmed that it does grow in several localities in the county. Its best-known use was as a cosmetic preparation for the skin.

CUCKOO FLOWER or **LADIES' SMOCK** (G. *biolair ghriagain*; L. *Cardamine pratense*)
Like many cresses this was considered good for reducing fevers and curing scurvy. It also had a reputation for soothing epileptic fits.

DAISY (G. *neòinean* [common daisy], *an neònan mòr* [gowan, ox-eye daisy]; L. *Bellis perennis* [common], *Chrysanthemum leucanthemum* [gowan])
The flowers of daisies, as well as those of narrow and broad-leaved plantain, were believed to be good for ophthalmic conditions, and the daisy plant was mixed into an ointment for cuts and bruises. The gowan, or ox-eye daisy, was sometimes made into a tea to treat asthma. Its juice boiled with honey was drunk for coughs, and the same preparation was applied externally for wounds.

*DANDELION (G. *am beàrnan Brìghde* [the notched plant of Brigid]; L. *Taraxacum leontodon*)
The dandelion was sacred to the goddess Brigid. An infusion of the root, sometimes the whole herb, was a highly regarded stomach tonic, especially for promoting appetite in cases of tuberculosis, (see also CENTAURY, GENTIAN and other bitters). Barbara Fairweather says

in *Highland Plant Lore* that dandelion leaves between bread and butter were an old cure for ulcers in Glencoe village, and also that coffee was traditionally made in the district from the dried and ground roots.

Norman Macdonald notes in the *Journal of Scandinavian Folklore* that the juice from the boiled roots was taken for internal pains in general.[11] The fresh plant juice was commonly used, more latterly in children's lore, to remove warts. It is no more or less effective in this than many other wart cures but it has a dramatic advantage – the white juice turns the skin black, though only transiently.

DOCKEN or **DOCK** (G. *copag*; L. *Rumex obtusifolius*, and several other species not distinguished in vernacular usage)
Sometimes used in place of the **BOGBEAN**, q.v. A decoction taken internally was said to be good for scurvy. Water dock was used for cleaning the teeth.

In Badenoch the thick root stock was cleaned and peeled, then the fibrous tissue was crushed into a pulp and made into a poultice to relieve bee or nettle stings. Writing of the good sense of this, Alexander McCutcheon remarks: 'The large percentage of water in the root, kept in suspension by the albuminous matter, has a soothing and cooling effect upon the inflamed surface, which by the slow evaporation of the water is continued for a considerable time. The poultice was kept on for about four or six hours, and repeated until the swelling and inflammation had disappeared.'[12]

In Lochaber a healing ointment was made by boiling docken roots until soft and mixing with equal parts of beeswax and fresh homemade butter.

*ELDER (G. *ruis*; L. *Sambucus nigra*)
Elder flowers and birch bark were boiled together in spring water which was strained off and drunk as a tonic. Elderflower water also

made a good skin tonic. The leaves were crushed into an ointment for wounds and burns. A fungus growing on its bark made a useful gargle for sore throats. The powdered bark made a laxative. Elderberry tea or wine was reckoned one of the best remedies for colds, flu and chest complaints like asthma and bronchitis.

Máire Black, who was brought up in the west of Ireland, and now lives in Scotland, remembers how as a child she helped to collect elder flowers for an ointment which her father made. The children were told that it was very important to hold something under the flowers being gathered so that the pollen would be saved. The flowers and pollen were taken up to the house and boiled in almond oil and lard. 'It smells horrible,' she said, 'but can be used for any skin conditions – eczema, chapped skin and so on – though not for cuts or wounds.' Her mother always used it as face cream, and they all used it to remove greasepaint after school plays. If applied quickly enough after being stung by nettles, it would even prevent the weals appearing. It was also a protective. 'People kept writing to ask for a jar, or coming to the door for one', said Máire.

*ELDER, dwarf or ground (G. *lus an easbaig*; L. *Aegopodium podagraria*) Once cultivated and used in cases of gout. A poultice of the crushed plant was used for sciatica. (It is also known in English as goat- gout- or bishop-weed).

*EYEBRIGHT (G. *lus nan leac, glanruis*; L. *Euphrasia officinalis*) Decoctions made from the common eyebright, milk, and cold tea were used as eyewashes. One method was to infuse the plant in milk then apply the liquid to the patient's eye with a feather.

FENNEL (G. *lus an t-saoidh*; L. *Foeniculum vulgare*) The Beatons recommended fennel for increasing the flow of urine.

*FERNS (G. *raineach*; L. *Filocopsida* – and see under separate species)
An unspecified bruised fern was mixed with white of egg as an application for inflamed eyes. **Hart's tongue fern**, (G. *creamh na muice fiadhaich* [wild pig's garlic]; L. *Asplenium scolopendrium*), was made into an ointment for burns. **Male fern** (G. *marc-raineach*; – L. *Dryopteris filix-mas*) was useful for worming. **Common polypody** G. *clach raineach*; L. *Polypodium vulgare*) was made into a medicine for catarrh. Decoctions of **spleenwort** (G. *dubhchasach* [for both maidenhair and black spleenwort]; L. *Asplenium*, various species) were given to people suffering from tuberculosis and spleen disorders.

Perhaps the most intriguing cure was made from the **royal fern** (G. *raineach rìoghail*; L. *Osmunda regalis*) and used to treat a dislocated knee pan. The roots of the young royal fern were gathered and chopped up, then put in a pan where they were covered with water. After the pot had boiled for a while on the fire, and then cooled sufficiently, the contents were applied to the injured knee and, according to the Revd Norman Macdonald, 'forthwith the pain stopped, all swelling disappeared and the kneecap went back to its original place'.

Royal fern spores were among a number of pollen remains found in several Stone Age sherds unearthed by archaeologist Caroline Wickham-Jones in the island of Rum in the 1980s. Investigations by archaeo-botanist Dr Brian Moffat found that the mix of plant remains was the likely residue of heather ale. The presence of royal fern puzzled him until he discovered that it would have been used as an agent for halting fermentation.

FIGWORT (G. *torranan, lus nan cnapan*; L. *Scrofularia nodosa*)
Used as an infusion for scrofulous diseases and an application for piles.
See under **TORRANAN** below, for discussion.

*FIR CLUB MOSS (G. *garbhag an t-sléibhe*; L. *Lycopodium selago, L. clavatum*)

An infusion of the moss was widely used as a skin tonic by women and girls. I first learned of it from an elderly woman who spent her childhood in west Sutherland at the beginning of this century. She and her brothers and sisters were regularly sent by their mother to collect large amounts of a moss they knew in Gaelic as *garbhag an t-sléibhe*, 'the little rough (or, perhaps, thick) one of the moors'. When the children returned with their haul, their mother would steep the moss in a big pot of boiling water which would be left to simmer for a while. The liquid was then strained off, left to cool, and used as a soothing and softening lotion for the women's and girls' faces, arms and hands.

Pliny names this moss as one of the most important herbs of the druids, and remarks on their curious method of gathering it. It was not to be touched with iron, and the gatherer had to pluck it by stealth and surprise, with his right hand thrust through the left armhole of his garment. His clothing had to be white and his feet freshly washed and bare. Immediately before the gathering, a sacrificial offering of bread and wine was made.

My informant died several years before I came across Pliny's description, but I think we can take it that those early twentieth-century children were not quite so fussy. They did, however, have one caution – the moss must be taken home in a scrupulously clean cloth.

The druids believed the moss should be carried as an amulet against fatal accidents, and that its smoke was good for eye diseases. Highland women used an infusion of this plant as an emetic and emmenagogue, but it needed to be used with caution. Its action can be violent and unless taken in very small doses the purging can cause some nasty side-effects.

FLAG, yellow (G. *seilistear*; L. *Iris pseudacorus*).
Snuff made from its roots helped to relieve colds. In Mull and some other places, the root was used as a cure for toothache and inflamed

throats. A nutmeg-sized piece of the root was bruised in a mortar with a handful of daisies, then the juice was strained through a linen cloth and a teaspoonful poured into each of the patient's nostrils. 'This strange application', noted Lightfoot, in 1777, 'is immediately followed by a kind of salivation, or copious defluxion of rheum from the mouth and nostrils, which often effects a cure, but not without great danger of the patient's taking cold during the violence of the operation.'[13]

FLAX (G. *lìon*; L. *Linum usitatissimum*)
A linseed poultice was applied as a general cure for any kind of swelling and was considered especially useful in drawing pus.

FLAX, fairy (G. *lìon na mnà* [or *ban*] *sìthe, lus mìosach* [menstrual plant] or *lus caolach*; L. *Linum catharticum*)
A dangerous plant if used by unskilled people, it was used mainly for gynaecological and menstrual problems. It was also a violent purge.

FOXGLOVE (G. *lus nam bansìth* [fairy women's plant]; L. *Digitalis purpurea*)
In Gaelic traditional medicine the use of foxgloves as a remedy for dropsy (fluid swellings which can be a symptom of certain cardiac problems) probably followed in the wake of Dr William Withering's famous discovery of an English folk cure for the problem in 1785. In the Highlands foxgloves were more generally used for a variety of other conditions.

A direct application of the moistened leaves to the skin proved a valuable remedy for the 'rose' (G. *ròs*) – a term which covered any erythematous condition of the skin, from simple erythema and eczema to true erysipelas. Foxglove leaves were also considered an excellent application for boils.

An old woman in Kilmonivaig, Inverness-shire made the following cure from a recipe she had from her mother and which is preserved in a hand-written note at the Highland Folk Museum, Kingussie: 'For a man in great pain from internal growth or swelling, a pulp was made from squashed foxglove roots, then applied inside flannel, after the pulp had been heated, as a poultice to the swelling. The man received immediate relief, and continued to do so until the cure was completed.'[14]

In the Braes of Lochaber chopped foxglove leaves and butter and garlic or onion heated were deemed 'good for drawing things, good for bad knees and for diphtheria – as a poultice on the knees, neck, and so on'.[15]

*GARLIC, wild (G. *creamh*; L. *Allium ursinum*)
The Gaels of old were rather partial to garlic and the wild variety was abundant in many areas. Older people living today in the wooded Sleat area of Skye tell how their mothers would use *creamh* as a pot herb. Infused on its own and taken internally for the 'stone', it was a popular cure, and it was also deemed very good for purifying and strengthening the blood. Alone or with other ingredients it was often made into a 'drawing' poultice.

GEAN or wild cherry (G. *geanais*; L. *Prunus avium*)
A tissane of the stalks made an astringent drink, and the gum, dissolved in wine, was used for colds.

GENTIAN (G. *lus a' chrùbain*; L. *Gentiana campestris*)
The Gaelic name for the field gentian came about because it was once mainly used in a cattle ailment called *an crùban*, a term which means

'croodling' (explained by Angus MacFarlane as 'The feet of the animal [being] so affected that the hind feet and the fore feet are drawn towards each other.'

Humans took internal infusions for indigestion and as a stomach tonic. (See also **CENTAURY** and other bitters.)

GERMANDER SPEEDWELL (G. *nuallach*; L. *Veronica chamaedrys*)
The pre-Linnaean Latin name of this plant was *Betonica Pauli* and this designation in old writings has sometimes led to its confusion with wood betony. It was a highly valued vulnerary among the Gaels and combined with herbs such as St John's wort to make an ointment for wounds. It also appears to have had a magically protective significance.

The West Highland Museum in Fort William has in its collection a hussif containing a letter which says '. . . I send a small bag, if you should chance to go to Battle or an [affair?] of honour, it will be no trouble to put it Round your Neck. I trust it will save you from Your Enemy.' Stitched into the letter is a small square of satin, pebbles, seeds, pieces of stalk and a tiny padlock. The seeds have been identified as those of either the germander or mountain speedwell, the latter being a species found mainly, if not exclusively, in the Scottish Highlands. The letter was sent to Colonel John Cameron of Fassifern (on the north side of Loch Eil) who, despite the charm, fell at Quatre Bras on the eve of the battle of Waterloo in 1815.

It is likely that the 'betony tea' mentioned by some sources as having been popular is the north Highlands was, in fact, made from germander speedwell once commonly used for making a tea in Sweden.[16]

GOLDEN ROD (G. *fuinnseag coille*; L. Solidago virgaurea)
For wounds, an ointment was made of St John's wort, germander speedwell, and golden rod cut small and mixed in butter and grease.

In a variation, the golden rod was mixed with all-heal and fresh butter. It was also believed to heal broken bones.

GOOSEBERRY (G. *gròsaid*; L. *Ribes grossularia*)

The prickles were used as charms to remove warts and styes. A wedding ring was laid over the wart and pricked through the ring with a gooseberry thorn. Ten such thorns were plucked, the other nine simply being pointed at the part affected, and then thrown over the shoulder.

GROUND IVY (G. *iadhshlat thalmhainn*; L. *Nepeta glechoma*)

In some parts a tea was made from ground ivy, sweetened with honey, and taken two or three times a day for consumption and coughs. Snuff was made from the dried leaves and used for asthma and headaches. Tradition has it that it was excellent for snake bites.

GROUNDSEL (G. *am bualan;* L. *Senecio vulgaris*)

A cataplasm of groundsel was said to be excellent for boils. The groundsel was washed, laid in a basin, and boiling water poured over it. Then it was covered and left to steam a little. Some of the water was poured off and put to 'foment' the boil. Then the cataplasm, or poultice, of groundsel was applied and covered to keep in the warmth. The poultice was renewed as necessary. Alternatively, the groundsel was applied cold to act as a coolant on a swelling or bruise, or inflamed or hardened breasts. A lotion for chapped hands was made by pouring boiling water over the plant and applying the liquid that was strained off.

HAWTHORN (G. *sgiach*, *sgitheach*; L. *Crataegus monogyna*)

Flowers and leaves made a decoction for sore throats. Hawthorn tea was also a 'balancer' for either high or low blood pressure.

*HEATHER (G. *fraoch*; L. *Calluna vulgaris*, and *Erica* – various species)

In 1582 the Scots historian George Buchanan remarked on the healthy Highland custom of using heather shoots for bedding:

> In this manner they form a bed so pleasant, that it may vie in softness with the finest down, while in salubrity it far exceeds it; for heath, naturally possessing the powers of absorption, drinks up the superfluous moisture, and restores strength to the fatigued nerves, so that those who lie down languid and weary in the evening, arise in the morning vigorous and sprightly.[17]

As a poultice for insomnia, heather was sometimes applied to the head long after it had gone out of fashion as a bedding material. Some of the older people still put sprigs of it under their pillows. Buchanan was right, even a heather pillow will give a refreshing sleep and an occasional cup of heather tea does wonders for the 'nerves'. People used to drink heather ale as a tonic and it is a custom that would be none the worse of a revival. Tubercular patients were given a decoction made from flowering heather tops.

HELLEBORINE (G. *ealabor geal*; L. *Epipactis latifolia*)

Snuff made from white helleborine was said to be good for the common cold.

*HERB ROBERT (G. *lus an ròis*; L. *Geranium Robertum*)

It was believed at one time to be a potent remedy for erysipelas and skin cancer. A man in the Lochend district of Inverness-shire was still prescribing it in the 1920s, and maintained he had cured several people with it.

The Kingussie pharmacist, Alexander McCutcheon, wrote in 1919:

> Herb Robert, or *lus an Eallain* or *Righeal Cùil*, to give it its Gaelic names [presumably for the Badenoch area], was a very popular remedy and highly spoken of. The Gaelic means 'plant for the hives', thus indicating its remedial properties. The entire plant was cut up into small pieces, and infused for about an hour in boiling water. Two ounces of the plant gave one imperial pint of infusion. The dose was adjusted according to the age of the patient, but no maximum dose is mentioned, and apparently it varied according to use and wont. It is difficult to tell why such a pungent-smelling plant received such glowing approbation, but despite its odorous drawbacks, its reputation as a 'certain cure' still remains.[18]

*HONEYSUCKLE (G. *féithlean*; L. *Lonicera periclymenum*)
The flowers were crushed and infused in boiling water to make a tea for relieving the symptoms of asthma and bronchitis. It was said the druids used honeysuckle to heal disorders of the eyes. It was also used to make a wash for getting rid of freckles or soothing sunburnt skin. Honeysuckle tea was believed to be a useful remedy for nervous headaches.

HOREHOUND (G. *gràbhan bàn*; L. *Marrubium vulgare*)
Horehound tea was popular for bronchitis and asthma, and McCutcheon said it was the specific remedy for coughs of all kinds:

> The whole plant, in the proportion of four ounces to an imperial pint of boiling water, was infused for some time and the demulcent liquid given as a drink. A sharp distinction was made between a cough and a cold. A cough was not considered serious, and the sick person

followed his usual vocation. A cold was totally different. The invalid was kept in bed and given oatmeal gruel, with butter, salt, and pepper, as well as spruce beer (a fermented solution of molasses and spruce twigs), to reduce the fever. It was not until all feverish symptoms had disappeared that any attention was given to the cough. The demulcent drink, prepared from the common white horehound, was given a truly excellent hygienic method of treatment.[19]

HORSETAIL (G. *clois*; L. *Equisetum arvense*)
Water in which the plant had been simmered provided a wash for wounds. The plant itself was used for scouring pots and pans.

HOUSELEEK (G. *lus nan cluas*; L. *Sempervivum tectorum*)
The literal translation of the Gaelic name is 'ear plant', and it was so-called because its juice, sometimes mixed with cream, was used as a cure for earache and deafness. The houseleek had many medicinal uses and was said to have been particularly good for soothing shingles and burns as well as cooling fevers. If it grew on a roof it was supposed to shield a house from fire and lightning. Its reputation in medicine is ancient and it is linked with legends throughout Europe.

IVY (G. *eidheann*; L. *Hedera helix*)
Highlanders, like many other country people, had long used the leaves, soaked in vinegar, as medication for corns. An ointment made from the leaves was used also for burns, and the twigs were boiled in butter as a salve for sunburn.

JUNIPER (G. *samhan, aiteann*; L. *Juniperis communis*)
This plant was the Gaels' cure for dropsy. It was also used as a stimulant and an ingredient of lotions and ointments. Its berries were used for

flavouring drinks and making astringents. A poultice of bruised juniper berries was said to be very good for snakebites.

LADY'S MANTLE (G. *copan an driùchd, trusgan* [A. alpina]; L. *Alchemilla vulgaris, A. alpina*)
Known better in southern herbals as a 'woman's herb', lady's mantle was used more commonly in the Highlands as an application for sores and wounds. The Gaelic name *copan an driùchd* means dew cup, a very exact description of the leaves which every morning hold a large and sparkling drop of dew in their centre.

LILY, White Water (G. *duilleag bhàite bhàn, bioras*; L. *Nymphaea alba*)
A curious use for this lovely plant was as a corn-remover. A recipe for this was sent me some years ago by Malcolm Macdonald, archivist to Argyll District Council, who came across it written on the back of an early eighteenth-century account in the Argyll papers at Inveraray Castle. Unfortunately the note is incomplete but enough of it has survived to tell of a fascinating old cure:

> Take roots of white Lillies so boyll them in winegar then make it like a plaister and Lay it on the Corne 3 or 4 dayes and night and it will make it fall of but the only thing in the world is a black snaill wrapte up in a Linnen Cloth laid before the fir and will rosted so bind it as hot as you cane enduer it to the corn and keep it supplied with fresh snals rosted 2 or 3 as need requers and it will make –

Under **SNAILS** and **SLUGS** in Chapter 12 it can be seen that these creatures are used to this day in cures for warts and corns. An added piece of interest is given to the Argyll prescription by virtue of the handwriting in the original. Ronald Black, cataloguer of Gaelic manuscripts in the National Library of Scotland, says that the writing is very similar to that of the Revd John Beaton, who died in 1712 and was the son of the last of the Mull physicians to practise under the old clan system.

*LOVAGE (G. *siunas, sunais*; L. *Ligusticum Scoticum*)
This plant of the sea-cliffs led something of a double life. Its daytime job was as a celery-like flavouring for broths and salads, but it moonlighted as a poor man's aphrodisiac. In lamb broth it was said to be 'very effectual' for people suffering from a trouble known as *glacach*, variously described as being a swelling in the palm of the hand or a form of consumption. The nourishing lamb and lovage broth is more likely to have been administered for the latter. Lovage was also eaten raw or served as a boiled vegetable with fish, meat or milk dishes.

Alistair Maclean's *Hebridean Altars*, which contains several interesting references to medicinal plants, has a tendency to put a rather utopian and pious gloss on everything, and lovage is no exception: '. . . they called [it] the Cajoler's Plant, since its soothing property gave quiet to the mind . . . ' However, lovage – as its English name implies – was a reputed aphrodisiac. Such was the reputation of its similarly endowed close cousin celery, that in medieval times Spanish nuns were forbidden to grow it in their convent gardens.

MARJORAM (G. *oragan, lus Mharsaili*; L. *Origanum vulgare*)
The plant was once very popular for making fomentations for stitches and other pains suffered by horses.

MERCURY, DOG'S (G. *lus Ghlinne Bhràcadail*; L. *Mercurialis perennis*)

Used as a powerful emetic and for cleaning wounds. Lightfoot says:

> It is called, in the ile of Skye, *Lus-glen-Bracadale*, and I was informed that it is there sometimes taken by way of infusion to bring on a salivation. How well it answers the intention I know not, but the experiment seems to be dangerous.[20]

MINT (G. *meannt*; L. *Mentha* – several species)
Before tea came into the country, dried mint was a favourite drink. Boiling water was poured over it in a pot in the same way as tea is infused. For a 'pain in the side after jaundice', which may have referred to a gall-bladder problem, boiled wild raspberry, wild mint and bogbean were given.

MISTLETOE (G. *uil'-ìoc*; L. *Viscum album*)
Mistletoe is rare in Scotland and flourishes only locally in a few places but the existence of alternative Gaelic names for it suggests that it was a familiar plant. Cameron's *Gaelic Names of Plants* gives, as well as the more widely known *uil'-ioc*, more of which later: *druidh-lus*, 'druid's herb'; *sùgh dharaich*, 'oak juice 'or substance'; and the Irish Gaelic *guis*, 'sticky'.

In 1772 Thomas Pennant wrote in his *Tour of Scotland* that country people gathered mistletoe and ivy, and kept them through the year to cure fevers and other troubles. This custom prevailed in Moray, where mistletoe is said to have grown on a tree near Elgin, well into the nineteenth century. Aside from fevers, it seems mainly to have been used to treat heart conditions and was taken as a general 'strengthener', though, as it is potentially poisonous, it would have taken a degree of skill to prepare remedial doses.

Since wild mistletoe is rare in Scotland, it may well have been specially grafted on to certain trees or bought from the pedlars who travelled all over the north and west Highlands selling fine china from the western English Midlands – where mistletoe flourishes – to even the humblest cottars. The plant is light and would have been relatively easy to carry about. By the 1890s remedies based on ivy and mistletoe were available in chemists' shops or via doctors' prescriptions – a viscum extract remains in the official pharmacopoeia to this day – and the practice of collecting the plants declined.

Dr Duncan Macgregor informed the Caledonian Medical Society at the end of the nineteenth century:

> When quite a lad, I distinctly remember an old woman in Inverness who used (when she could get it at the appropriate season) to make 'mistletoe tea'. When questioned as to why she did so, she would say that she felt the benefit from drinking it, as she suffered from palpitation of the heart. As may be imagined, no one believed it could really do her any good, and she was teased by everyone, obviously owing to the association of mistletoe and the heart. In all probability, however, the old woman told the truth, as 'viscum album' is now in every chemist's price list, and is looked upon as a substitute for digitalis.[21]

Roman writers noted that the druids' name for mistletoe was 'all-heal in their language', and the modern Gaelic *uil'-ìoc* literally translates 'all-heal'.

MONKSHOOD (G. *fuath a' mhadaidh* [wolf's bane]; L. *Aconitum napellus*)

An extremely poisonous plant, it was certainly employed by the Beaton physicians in the Middle Ages but needed great skill in administering the correct dose. It remains a common plant in many northern Highland gardens, especially in Sutherland. In Dingwall in 1856 three people, two priests and a landowner, were badly poisoned after having been served monkshood in mistake for horseradish, the roots of the plants being very similar.

*MUGWORT (G. *liathlus*; L. *Artemesia vulgaris*)
It was believed that travellers who carried mugwort would not tire. The plant has a bitter taste and is said to strengthen the stomach and create an appetite. In the Highlands the young, tender leaves were used as a pot herb. Before tobacco was imported, dried mugwort was a popular herb for smoking. In Scots the plant was known as 'muggins' and may have earned its place in the following rhyme from its use to treat anorexic young women.

> If they wad drink nettles in March and eat muggins in May,
> Sae many braw maidens wadna gang tae clay.

MUSTARD (G. *sgeallag*; L. *Sisymbrium officinale*)
It is likely that mustard cures became popular in the Highlands through the availability of the prepared powder, as it is not known to have been specifically cultivated in the area, although the wild mustard, charlock (in Gaelic *praiseach gharbh*), was used as a pot-herb.

A hot mustard bath is a well-known reliever and even preventive of the common cold throughout the British Isles but the Gael had a more sophisticated version that is well attested for its efficacy. Here is the method told to me by Ann MacDonell of Spean Bridge in Lochaber who, in turn, heard of it in her younger days from an elderly neighbour in Inver Roy: 'Put your feet in a hot mustard bath and drape a towel over the knees to keep in the steam for four or five minutes. Take a gill of whisky in toddy or gruel and jump into bed without drying your feet. Have plenty clothes on the bed and put fresh clothes on in the morning.' (For more dramatic variants on this, see Chapter 10.)

In pleurisy a mustard poultice was applied to the patient's side.

*NETTLE (G. *deanntag, feanntag*; L. *Urtica urens*)

The nettle had many uses in the old days. Cloth was woven from its fibres and it was eaten as a nourishing vegetable as well as being used in medicine where it was generally said to be good for the kidneys and urinary complaints, and for purifying the blood. There was an old belief that the plant grew from 'dead men's bones' and, indeed, it flourishes on the refuse left by humans – especially after urinating.

So far as I know, its use as a cure for insomnia was unique to the Highlands. For this, the nettle leaves were chopped very small and mixed with switched egg white. The mixture was then applied to the temples and forehead.

A decoction of the roots was given for tuberculosis and a nettle poultice was applied to minor cuts, grazes and wounds to stem the bleeding when the flow was not too great.

It was an important part of the spring diet and was often taken in the form of porridge or as a pot-herb to purify the blood after the winter. For *càl deanntaig*, nettle broth, the first tender shoots of the plant were minced and boiled and sometimes mixed with a little oatmeal. The broth was also taken for rheumatics, indigestion, coughs and as a general appetiser. It was recognised that only the very young shoots were suitable for eating but, as every frustrated gardener knows, if the plant is cut back, new shoots are generated throughout the summer.

OAK (G. *darach*; L. *Quercus robur*)

An infusion of the powdered bark was used as a gargle for sore throats.

*OAT (G. *corc*; L. *Avena sativa*)

Oatmeal, always kept in the house as part of the staple diet, was frequently resorted to for a remedy. For minor boils and suppurations an oatmeal poultice made with water and a slight dressing of salt butter was applied. For 'difficult' boils urine took the place of the butter.

In some places onions or soap and sugar were used instead of the butter and oatmeal poultice. In Lochaber there was great faith in applying the white in hen's dirt.

Oatmeal and butter was also used to alleviate hacks on the hands or feet. Common colds and coughs were treated with unsalted brochan, or water gruel, sweetened with honey and sometimes with the addition of butter.

Martin says: 'The Drink us'd at going to bed, disposeth one to sleep and sweat, and is very diuretick, if it hath no Salt in it.' The gruel was believed to be especially nourishing for consumptives.

A person could cure his own warts by taking eighty-one (nine times nine, a magical number) stems of oats, binding them into nine branches of nine each and secreting them under a stone; as the stems rotted, the warts were expected to disappear.

For sore eyes a handful of oatmeal was put into a bowl full of water, stirred, and left for a short time. The mixture was thoroughly strained through a cloth and the patient applied the meal water to his eyes. Oatmeal was also considered good for relieving colic.

*ONION (G. *uinnean*; L. *Allium cepa*)
For fever, a large red onion split in two, and hung one half at an open window and the other above the door, was thought useful in attracting a disease, as in a short time the onion assumed a soot-black colour.

For toothache a poultice of red onions was applied to the cheek. A mixture of chopped onions and seaweed was deemed an excellent 'drawing' application for a gathering when it was 'not coming on as quickly as it should do'.

In pneumonia two onions were boiled and an onion placed in each of the patient's armpits. For the reasoning behind this, see Chapter 3. Onions and/or garlic mixed with chopped foxglove leaves and butter made a highly regarded poultice for bad knees and diphtheria – in the latter the poultice was placed on the neck.

ORCHIDS

The twayblade orchid (G. *dà-dhuilleach*; L. *Listera ovata*), made an unusual but profitable Highland export in earlier centuries when it was a main ingredient in salep, a preparation for soothing irritated stomachs and bowels. Spotted orchid (G. *ùrach bhallach*; L. *Orchis maculata*) was sometimes used as a poultice for drawing small objects embedded in the flesh. In listing herbs for extracting foreign bodies Pliny gives the orchid for such wounds that have become infected. Almost all orchids were regarded as potent aphrodisiacs. This may derive from the shape of their roots but they also make an excellent, nourishing food which creates a sense of well-being. The early purple orchid was greatly esteemed as a demulcent – a soothing or protective lining for the alimentary canal.

PARSLEY (G. *pearsal*; L. *Carum petroselinum*)
Taken to increase urine flow.

PELLITORY, of Spain (G. *lus na Spainnte*; L. *Anthemis pyrethrum*)
Recommended for fevers.

PENNYROYAL (G. *peighinn rìoghail*; L. *Mentha pulegium*)
Infusions of bramble root and pennyroyal were given for bronchitis and asthma.

PEPPER (G. *peabar*; L. *Piper nigrum*)
I am assured that this was used to stop bleeding, though it surely cannot have been pleasant for the patient.

*PERIWINKLE, Lesser (G. *faochag*; L. *Vinca minor*)
The lesser periwinkle was used in an ointment for bruises and persistent skin irritations. Since modern investigations of the plant have found it useful in treating certain cancers, the esteem in which it was held in Highland medicine may have been derived from its efficacy in dealing with skin cancers. As in English, the Gaelic name *faochag* is used for both the plant and the shellfish.

PINE (G. *pin-chrann, giuthas* [Scots pine]; L. *Pinus* – various species)
In Badenoch an ointment was made from beeswax, hog's lard and resin, the later obtained from the trunks of various species of pine growing in the neighbourhood. The plaster was spread on linen in squares about four inches each way, and with a margin of about an inch. They were used for boils and sores. A plaster was warmed at the fire and applied to the boil, allowed to remain twelve hours, and then removed and burned; the part was then bathed and another plaster applied.

The bark of the pine, like that of a number of trees, is astringent and was used for agues.

*PLANTAIN (G. *cuach Phàdraig, slànlus*; L. *Plantago major, Plantago lanceolata*)
The leaves of the ribwort plantain (*slànlus; P. lanceolata*) were placed on cuts and those of the broad-leaved plantain (*cuach Phàdraig: P. major*) on 'gatherings', without a doubt as to their efficacy, said Dr H E Fraser of Inverness, at the end of the nineteenth century. Alexander McCutcheon adds: 'The entire leaves of the plantain were largely used in the fresh state as a styptic for small wounds and abrasions. The longest blades were taken and applied to the wound, and gave great relief, stopping the bleeding quickly.'[22]

Both narrow and broad-leaved plantain were thought to be remedies for ophthalmic conditions. In tonsillitis greater plantain leaves were applied externally to the throat. They were also said to be good for nettle stings and infected swellings.

If the skin was rubbed off the hand, or other part, ribwort leaves were moistened with saliva and rubbed on the part affected. It was said that a 'new skin was immediately (!) formed'.

The upper side of a leaf, whether mallow, ribwort, plantain, or any other, was always laid on a sore that was to be healed. The underside of a leaf was supposed to 'draw' a wound or sore, and was used to induce suppuration.

Fluxes (a term once applied to an increase in discharge from any bodily orifice) were treated with plantain which had been boiled in water in which a piece of red-hot quartz had been dropped.

POPPY, Common (G. *meilbheag*; L. *Papaver rhoeas*)
John Cameron, in *Gaelic Names of Plants*, says the juice was formerly put into children's food to make them sleep. In South Uist the flowers of the red poppy were made into a liquid to help with teething. The smoke from the yellow poppy was said to expel evil spirits.

POTATO (G. *buntàta*; L. *Solanum tuberosum*)
The humble tattie is proof of the adaptability of folk medicine. When the potato was first introduced into the Western Isles and Highlands in about 1739, Clanranald's people told him, when they lifted the first tubers, that although he could force them to grow such things, he need not expect them to eat them. Nevertheless, once the value of the crop was appreciated, the potato soon became a staple crop and by the end of the century it was widely grown throughout the country. By 1840, Dr Isabel Grant notes in her *Highland Folk Ways*,

potatoes were said to form three-quarters to seven-eighths of the food consumed by Highland families. As in Ireland, though not with quite such devastating consequences, the Highland potato famine of the late 1840s was a grim time.

It took no time at all for people to look to the tuber for likely remedies and by the early nineteenth century, if not before, it was an established part of the tradition and had even acquired quasi-magical properties, since there seems no other explanation for the strong belief that carrying a slice of raw potato in the pocket was a certain cure for rheumatism. 'I know, to this day,' said Dr Duncan Macgregor, who, in the last decade of the nineteenth century, was already referring to the use of the tattie as an 'old' Highland cure, 'people who thoroughly believe in this, and who assure you that they have never had a twinge of rheumatism since they commenced carrying the piece of potato, which statement may, of course, be true, though whether the potato has had to do with the immunity from the disease is another question.'[23]

A slice of potato was put on a black eye and for nose-bleeds a slice of raw potato was applied to the back of the neck.

PRIMROSE (G. *sòbhrag*; L. *Primula vulgaris*)
The leaves were used as a salve for burns and cuts. A native of Bernera, off the Isle of Lewis, Agnes Maclennan, remembers having persistent boils on her legs cured by an application of primrose leaves in the 1940s.

PUFFBALL (G. *caochag, balgann losgainn*; L. *Bovista nigrescens*)
The fine powder of the puffball formed an efficient haemostatic, provided there was not a profuse flow of blood and they were useful in the treatment of piles. When young, that is before they ripen and the flesh starts to discolour, they may be eaten. Long ago people used the smoke from the burning, mature, puffball, to stupefy wild bees

in order to collect the honey. There was a belief that the spores could cause blindness, which may have resulted from the fact that the spores can have an anaesthetic effect if inhaled in quantity. Sliced mushrooms were applied to burns and scalds.

QUEEN OF THE MEADOW or MEADOWSWEET (G. *crios Chu-Chulainn*; L. *Filipendula ulmaria*)

Pennant lists meadowsweet among treatments for flux which included 'jelly of bilberry, or a poultice of flour and suet; or new churned butter; or strong cream and fresh suet boiled, and drunk plentifully morning and evening'. Traditionally used for treating fevers and headaches, its Gaelic name, meaning Cu-Chulainn's belt, comes from a story about the great Celtic hero. Ill with a fierce fever, Cu-Chulainn was cured by being bathed in meadowsweet.

In South Uist meadowsweet was used for reducing fevers and long ago it was sometimes used as a floor-covering along with bog-myrtle and fleabane – a more easily changed, hygienic and fragrant cover than our modern carpeting.

RASPBERRY (G. *preas sùbh chraobh*; L. *Rubus idaeus*)

A light dish of boiled wild raspberry, wild mint and bogbean was given after jaundice. Highland women also used the widely known raspberry-leaf tea therapy to strengthen the muscles of the womb before giving birth. In Skye the juice was added in syrup form to punches. Distilled raspberry water was given as a cooling drink to feverish patients.

RHUBARB (G. *luibh na purgaid*; L. *Rheum rhaponticum*)

'Itchiness in the flesh' was treated by seven doses of stewed rhubarb. It was said that relief came to the patient before he ate the seventh dose . . .

ROSE (G. *ròs, mucag* [haw]; L. *Rosa* – various species)
Decoctions of rose wood and leaves, with poultices of the leaves
and fresh butter locally, were used in conjunction with infusions of
stonecrop or herb Robert (taken internally) to treat erysipelas, a
condition itself known as the 'rose'.

*ROWAN (G. *caorann*; L. *Sorbus aucuparia*)
A good gargle can be made from the berries by boiling them to a
pulp, then they should be squeezed through muslin and strained for
use. Whooping cough was relieved with a decoction of apples and
rowanberries sweetened with brown sugar. Lightfoot mentions that
in Jura 'they use the juice of [the rowan] as an acid for punch'.

RUE, Lesser meadow or alpine (G. *rù beag*; L. *Thalictrum minus or
T. alpinus*)
Infusions of rue were given for worms. The lesser meadow rue, *T.
minus*, was a powerful cathartic.

*SAGE (G. *sàiste*; L. *Salvia officinalis*)
Wild sage chewed and put into the ears of cows or sheep was
considered certain to restore eyesight; chopped small and mixed with
oats, it was used for worming horses.
    An old Latin saying about the sage is given in Gaelic as:

> *Carson a gheibheadh duine bàs*
> *Aig am bheil sàiste fàs 'na ghàradh?*

Why should a man die that has sage growing in his garden? runs
the English version. For some reason (herbal correctness, perhaps?)

hardly any modern writers on plants add the astute old answer: Because no herb that grows in the garden is strong enough to fight death.

*ST JOHN'S WORT (G. *lus* or *achlasan Chaluim Chille*; L. *Hypericum perforatum*, *H. pulchrum*)
A favourite amulet if the plant is come across without being specifically sought, *achlasan Chaluim Chille* means the 'armpit package of St Columba' and thereby, needless to say, hangs a tale (told in Chapter 3). It is one of the oldest known Highland cures, and one of the most valuable. An ointment of St John's wort, germander speedwell and golden rod chopped and mixed in butter and grease was considered the very best application for wounds. In Glen Roy where the plant is known in Gaelic as *lus na fala*, 'bloodwort', St John's wort was boiled to stem bleeding.

SANICLE, Wood (G. *bodan coille*; L. *Sanicula Europaea*)
Used externally and internally as an astringent and vulnerary, this plant was especially important in the traditional medicine of the Western Isles, for healing infected wounds and ulcers.

SCABIOUS (G. *ura bhallach*; L. *Scabiosa succisa*)
The root was applied for the relief of toothache and the itch.

SCURVY-GRASS (G. *am maraiche, carran, plàigh na carra*; L. *Cochlearia officinalis*)
This small, fleshy-leaved plant which grows near the shore was not only gathered from the wild but also cultivated. Fairweather says that it was reckoned to be taken at breakfast as late as the nineteenth

century. As well as being eaten as an important anti-scorbutic it was also made into a useful poultice for boils or cramps.

It was popular among sailors and fishermen and it is likely that it was used by Viking seafarers on their longer voyages. It is interesting that the Gaelic name *am maraiche* means 'the sailor'. Scurvy-grass was also considered good for the stomach.

*SEAWEED (G. *feamainn*; L. *alga* – general terms, individual names are given below)
Seaweeds of various kinds held an important place in the Gaelic materia medica and daily diet, its iodine content being particularly valuable.

The type which Martin (and several other commentators, perhaps influenced by Martin) call 'linarich' is probably the *lùireach* (literally, cloak, which in miniature it resembles when fresh; when dried out along the lower shore and on rocks it forms papery thin, irregular sheets) referred to by the Revd Norman Macdonald:

> In mid and late summer, after a prolonged period of dry sunny weather, one will come across among the dried seaweed and shingle on the beach, strips of filmy, skinlike, form of seaweed, called lùireach in Gaelic. I have never heard the English term for it, nor have I come across the Gaelic word itself as applied to a seaweed or marine substance, in print. Anyway, the lùireach was collected and baked on an iron griddle, over a fire. It was then placed over the goitre and left there, a bandage having been tied round it to keep it from shifting. I have heard of one patient who was to undergo a surgical operation for goitre. A short time before he was due to enter hospital, he was advised by an old Highland woman, to try the lùireach cure, which he did with complete success. The goitre vanished and he did not have to go to hospital.[24]

'Linarich, a green-coloured seaweed, was applied to the temples and forehead for bleeding from the nose', notes a doctor in the Caledonian Medical Journal for 1896.[25] Martin describes what appears to be a type of sea lettuce (*Ulva lactuca or the Monostroma grevillei*) thus:

> Linarich, a very thin small Plant, about eight, ten, or twelve inches in length; it grows on Stone, on Shells, and on the bare Sand. The Plant is apply'd Plaister-wise to the Forehead and Temples, for removing the Megrim, and also to Heal the Skin after a Clister-Plaister of Flammula Jovis [Spearwort].[26]

Slake (G. *slòcan*; L. *Porphyra umbilicalis*), known in Ireland as 'sloke' and in Wales as 'laver', was eaten boiled and dressed with butter and it was claimed that a person might live on slake and butter alone without any bread or other nourishment and at the same time undertake any heavy labour. It is similar in form to the sea lettuce but a much darker, purplish colour.

Seaweed was also considered highly effective for rheumatism. For 'rheumatics in the knee' knotted seaweed was cooked on an iron griddle over the fire. The hot seaweed was then placed over the knee and tied with a bandage. Channelled fucus (G. *feamainn chìrean*; L. *fucus canaliculatus*), a short crisp seaweed found near high water mark, boiled in sea water, was also found very effective when applied to a rheumaticky knee.

When skin disorders and eruptions were found to be caused by general ill health, an excellent remedy was found in dulse soup, taken two or three times a week, or more often. Dulse soup was still a favourite dish in some parts of the Highlands in the 1960s and it is a pity that so many old recipes are out of fashion because of the convenience of easier-to-prepare shop-bought provisions. Sometimes a dish of boiled dulse was simply prepared with butter. Dulse soup, *càl duilisg*, was believed to be one of the best remedies for indigestion and stomach disorders in general. While dulse (G. *duileasg*; L. *Palmaria palmata*) could be eaten raw, and helped to ward off hunger when working on the shore, it was much more palatable and digestible when cooked.

In the islands it was eaten raw to improve eyesight and relieve constipation – though it was said to be more effective for the latter if taken boiled and the juice drunk with it. Like 'linarich' it was applied in a plaster to the temples to relieve migraine; for colic and stone it was boiled and eaten in its own juice; and for worming it was dried without washing (not perhaps such a good idea in these more polluted times), powdered and taken after fasting.

Dulse had a great reputation for helping to evacuate the after-birth. For this purpose an amount of the fresh weed was applied externally to the lower abdomen.

The 'blade' of the sea-tangle (G. *stamh*; L. *Laminaria digitata*), which was to become an important part of the short-lived island kelp industry, was also edible and Martin tells the story of a young man who had lost his appetite and who was advised to boil the blade and drink the infusion with a little butter. The patient's condition, which failed to respond to the orthodox pills of the day, was soon restored to a healty state.

Seaweeds were also among the numerous substances used in the Highlands as 'drawing' applications for difficult boils and gatherings. In the *Caledonian Medical Journal*, Dr Duncan Macgregor says that 'Seaweed was looked upon as a sovereign cure for "thickneck" and other swellings, not doubt rightly so, owing to the iodine which it contained.'[27]

A condition often mentioned in old Gaelic medical references is 'falling of the uvula'. So dreaded was it that it even had its own preventive charm – a piece of a small red seaweed found in pools of water when the tide is out, tied with a piece of cord, and carried about the person of the patient. It had to be gathered by some other person, who said, while handing it over to the patient – '*Ann an ainm an Athar, a' Mhic, agus an Spioraid Naoimh, air cioch-shlugain AB.*') In the name of the Father, Son and Holy Ghost, for the uvula of AB).

Carrageen (G. *an cairgein* L. *Chondus crispus*) was gathered at the very low waters of the equinoctial tides and laid out in rain and sun for natural washing and bleaching. It could then be stored for use throughout the rest of the year. I have used it in stews, puddings and fruit jellies where it is a very effective and nourishing thickening or setting agent with a delicate flavour. In the old days it was used for the same purposes, especially for thickening milk or cream, and as a valuable diet for invalids.

SHEPHERD'S PURSE (G. *sporan* or *lus na fala*; L. *Capsella bursa-pastoris*)
For open wounds and haemorrhages.

SILVERWEED (G. *brisgean, barr brisgein*; L. *Potentilla anserina*)
The tuberous roots were sometimes eaten raw, especially by children, and had a rough nutty flavour. When roasted the nutty flavour was rather more subtle and pleasant. The dried or roasted root could be ground into a type of flour.

It is possible that before cereals were first cultivated in the Highlands, about 4000 BC, silverweed meal may have been part of the staple diet. As late as the eighteenth century it was much resorted to in some of the islands in times of famine. During the Clearances it became a useful foodstuff for the dispossesseed, since it is one of the few edible plants that sheep abhor.

SLOE (G. *àirneag*; L. *Prunus spinosa*)
Sloe jelly was used for a relaxed throat. The flowers made into an infusion were used externally for scabies. A decoction of the root and bark was used for asthma.

SNEEZEWORT (G. *luibh bhàn*; L. *Achillaea ptarmica*)
The boiled juice was taken for stomach troubles.

SOUROCK or **SORREL** (G. *samh, sealbhad, puinneag, puinneagan*; L. *Rumex acetosa*, and other varieties)

The leaf, which has a sharp, sour taste, was sometimes chewed to relieve thirst when out on the hill or by children out at play. As a cooling herb it was sometimes given in infusions to fever patients or used as an appetiser. It was a well-reputed remedy for healing minor wounds and bruises, and belongs to the same family (*Rumex*) as docken and a number of other medical herbs. Common sorrel was eaten for tuberculosis.

Dog sorrel, *sealbhag nan con*, was eaten as a salad and reckoned more succulent than sheep's sorrel. Mountain sorrel (L. *Oxyria digyna*), known in Gaelic as *sealbhag nam fiadh* (literally deer sorrel), is salty as well as acidic in taste.

SPEARWORT (G. *glas-leum* or *lasair-theine*; L. *Flammula jovis, Ranunculus flammula*)

Spearwort, also known as spirewort or spinewort, was bruised, placed in a limpet shell and applied to the jaw to relieve toothache, a fairly drastic resort as it was also used to raise blisters. This was sometimes used by the poorer people instead of cantharides (Spanish fly) to raise blisters.

SPHAGNUM MOSS (G. *còinneach dhearg*; L. *Sphagnum Cymbifolium*)

Widely used as a dressing for wounds and women's periods as well as the forerunner of the disposable nappy, this ubiquitous moss of the bogs was easily gathered, picked clean of foreign material and left to dry in the sun. When dry it was not only highly absorbent but also mildly antiseptic. Its use for field dressings from the Napoleonic wars onwards is believed to have been prompted by the initiative of Highland soldiers when regulation-issue dressings were scarce. During the

First and Second World Wars sphagnum moss was gathered in many areas of the Highlands and sent for processing in the south as a basis for dressings.

Whether soliders employed it for march-weary feet, I do not know, but it was certainly used for sore feet in the Highlands, where, as well as alder leaves, formentations of warm water in which sphagnum had been simmered made a popular rub for travellers' weary limbs before going to bed.

SPURGE, Petty (G. *lus-leighis*; L. *Euphorbia peplus*)
The caustic, milky-looking juice of this plant was commonly used to destroy warts in many European folk traditions. Otherwise the petty spurge was, justifiably, looked upon as an extremely poisonous plant fit only for occasional use as a violent purge, and then only in very small doses. Why then did the Gaels single it out for the distinctive and honoured name of *lus leighis*, the 'healing herb' when they were so well versed in the remedial properties of a wealth of plants at their disposal, many of which might have vied for the title? This species of Euphorbia has recently been clinically investigated for its use in cancer treatments, and it is my guess that its usefulness in healing skin cancers was recognised centuries ago by the Gaelic physicians. When more of their medieval manuscripts come to be translated, we may learn the answer.

STONECROP (G. *gràbhan nan clach*; L. *Sedum acre*)
An infusion was used to treat the 'rose' (erysipelas).

TANSY (G. *lus na Frainge*; L. *Tanacetum vulgare*)
Depending on the degree of the problem, and the general health of the patient, varying strengths of tansy tea were administered for

worms. Sometimes the tansy was infused in whey and whisky. It was always taken while fasting, which usually meant a dose first thing in the morning.

TEA

In the old days tea meant an infusion of any refreshing herb, but in the Highlands as elsewhere the introduction of the dried leaves of the *Camellia thea* led to it alone being referred to as 'tea' proper and any other kind being put to one side as a 'herbal tea', as if, somehow, the camellia herb was the acceptable grocery item and all the rest mere quaint museum pieces.

Even when tea was still very dear during the eighteenth and most of the nineteenth centuries, the poorest Gaels made sacrifices to afford this splendid herb which was to become to the cup what the tattie so quickly became to the plate. Because of its high cost in early days – at the end of the eighteenth century tea cost from five to seven shillings a pound at a time when a single sheep sold for between three and a half to eight shillings – tea was usually taken only in the evenings. At the end of the nineteenth century it was still common for Highland people to eke out their supply by adding other herbs. For example, half a teaspoon of tea with an equal amount of caraway seed might be infused for two people. Later, other herbal or spicy ingredients were added simply for the taste. One of my neighbours, Mary Mackay, who is in her mid-eighties, still keeps cloves in her tea caddy and occasionally adds a touch of nutmeg to her teapot, a custom she inherited from her own mother. She serves the tea black and sugarless and it is delicious.

THISTLE (G. [generally] *giogan, cluaran*; L. *Compositae family*)
The bulbous heads of some thistles were cut, placed on a flat stone and broken open by pounding with another stone. The inside was sweet

and good for chewing. Children especially sought it out as a 'sweet'. Thistle tea was claimed to dispel depression and melancholy.

THYME (G. *Lus an rìgh*, 'king's herb'; L. *Thymus serpyllum*)
Thyme was considered one of the most potent of tonics, especially for the nerves and weak chests. In the Western Isles wild thyme was put under the pillow or drunk as an infusion to prevent nightmares. Thyme tea was once popular throughout the Highlands as an everyday beverage. In areas where the lime-loving lavender did not grow well, women used flowering sprigs of thyme to scent their clothes, handkerchiefs and household linen.

TOBACCO (G. *tombaca*; L. *Nicotiana tabacum*)
Tobacco leaves were used in many areas to stop bleeding. During the world wars the actual tobacco plants were grown in some unlikely parts such as the stormy north coast of Sutherland where, when dried and cured, they apparently provided an acceptable smoke. For centuries, perhaps even millennia, prior to the introduction of tobacco, leaves from various native plants, such as betony and coltsfoot, were commonly smoked, latterly with the use of clay pipes. Mischievous children sometimes smoked peat dross – while not a pleasant experience it once did little to prevent them growing up with a taste for tobacco proper in the days before government health warnings. Where the leaf tobacco was not available for stemming bleeding the prepared variety was judged just as good, a plug of black twist being the most popular.

TORMENTIL (G. *leamhnach*; L. *Potentilla erecta*)
The dainty little yellow-flowered plant was used for worming. In Tiree and Coll a decoction of the roots in milk was given for diarrhoea and dysentery. In Uist it was chewed to heal a sore lip.

TORRANAN

'The *torranan*, a flowering plant growing on rocky hillsides, the bloom of which is large and pap-like, is also used as a charm for this purpose [against the effects of the Evil Eye], and is said to be very efficacious if culled during the flow of the tide,' Dr S Rutherford Macphail reported to the Caledonian Medical Society a hundred years ago.[28]

The various reports of this plant baffle me. It is a prime candidate for the sort of study urged at the start of this chapter. The most detailed account of it is given in *Carmina Gadelica*, but the flower described seems most like that of a wild carrot's full-blown umbel with its (occasional) central purplish floret resembling a nipple on a breast, while the root 'a cluster of four bulbs like the four teats of a cow' is something else. Carmichael translates *torranan* as 'figwort', yet this plant has rather insignificant dark red flowers although it has a nodular root.

VETCH, kidney (G. *meòir Mhoire, cas-an-uain*); L. *Anthyllis vulneraria*)
Found very useful as a balm for cuts and bruises.

*VETCH, tuberous (G. *carra-meille* or *carrachan*; L. *Lathyrus montanus* or *Orobus tuberosus*)
This plant's properties were highly esteemed by the Gaels and by the ancient Celts before them. I can confirm that its tubers taste every bit as good as the following description by the Revd. Angus MacFarlane claims:

> It has long, branching, underground roots, strung with nodulous lumps at frequent intervals. These, after they are dried, are chewed as wild liquorice. For chewing purpose I consider them superior to and far less deleterious than common chewing gum. The taste lingers

in the mouth for long after the last shred is chewed. They are said to ward off hunger for a long time. The taste is both acid and sweet, and never palls.[29]

In 1777 John Lightfoot wrote:

The Highlanders have a great esteem for the tubercles of the roots; they dry and chew them in general to give a better relish to their liquor; they also affirm them to be good against most diseases of the thorax, and that by the use of them they are enabled to repel hunger and thirst for a long time. In Breadalbane and Ross-shire they sometimes bruise and steep them in water, and make an agreeable fermented liquor with them. They have a sweet taste, something like the roots of liquorice, and when boiled, we are told, are well-flavoured and nutritive, and in times of scarcity have served as a substitute for bread.[30]

Thomas Pennant, too, sang its praises:

. . . among the useful plants, the Corr or Cor-meille must not be omitted, whose roots dried are the support of the highlanders in long journeys, amidst the barren hills destitute of the supports of life; and a small quantity, like the alimentary powders, will for a long time repel attacks of hunger. Infused in liquor it is an agreeable beverage, and, like the Nepenthe of the Greeks, exhilarates the mind. From the similitude of sound in the name, it seems to be the same with Chara, the root discovered by the soliders of Caesar at the siege Dyrrachium [de Bel. Civil Bk iii], which steeped in milk was such a relief to the famished army. Or we may reasonably believe it to have been the Caledonian food described by Dio [*Vita Severi*], of which the quanity of a bean would prevent both hunger and thirst: and this, says the historian, they have ready for all occasions.[32]

There seems no doubt that the plant referred to above as 'Chara' is the same as the one which gave its name to the Celtic and Gaelic 'nectar of the gods' named by other classical writers as the 'corma' (Athenaeus quoting Posidonius) or 'courmi' (Dioscurides) of the Celts, and in the early Gaelic literature of Ireland and Scotland as *cairm* or *cuirm*. In the Litany of *Aengus Céile Dé* (*c*. 798) a poem ascribed to St Brigid translates:

> I should like a great lake of ale [*corm*]
> For the king of kings;
> I should like the family of heaven
> To be drinking it through time eternal.

No apologies are made for writing and quoting about this plant at length since it has fallen into a strange neglect and, it seems to me, it is ripe for investigation and, perhaps, a revival if grown commercially. As late at the 1950s it was being gathered by older people in the north of Scotland for inclusion in a home-brewed heather ale. Now it is virtually unkown even by those with otherwise good memories of the old ways with plants.

One last quotation on the subject: Martin wrote of its use in Skye in the late seventeenth century:

> Carmel . . . has a blue Flower in July; the Plant itself is not us'd, but the Root is eaten to expel Wind: and they say it prevents Drunkenness, by frequent chewing of it; and being so us'd, gives a good Relish to all Liquors, Milk only excepted. It is Aromatick and the Natives prefer it to Spice for brewing Aquavitae; the Root will keep for many Years: some say that it is Cordial and allays Hunger.[32]

*VIOLET (G. *sail chuach*; L. *Viola odorata* (sweet violet) and *Viola canina* (dog violet)
Violets were used in a number of cures but one of their most popular uses among women was as a cosmetic. There was a saying:

Sail chuach is bainne ghabhar
Suath ri t'aghaidh
'S chan eil mac rìgh air an domhan
Nach bi air do dhéidh.

(Violets and goats' milk/Rub on your face/And there's no king's son in the world/That won't be after you.)

A decoction of the wood violet, bròg na cuthaid, in whey was considered useful in allaying fevers and the astringent leaves were applied for skin problems. The plant was also used in a decoction for headaches and catarrh.

*WATERCRESS (G. *biolair*; L. *Nasturtium officinalis*)

Watercress was commonly used for reducing fevers, and purifying and strengthening the blood. Because of the danger of liverfluke eggs, which are carried by sheep and often deposited on the plants, it is not safe to collect them where sheep are, or might have been, grazing. In Uist it is believed that if the cress is cut above the water line it will be safe to eat. At one time watercress formed a popular and nourishing part of the daily diet.

An old and solitary woman who survived the appalling massacre of her kin in 1577 when the Macleods of Harris herded the Macdonald islanders of Eigg into a cave and set a huge fire to its entrance, was told by the departing assassins that though she was spared the fire she would die slowly of hunger. The valiant woman is said to have called after them as they left in their boats: 'If I get shell-fish and dulse for my portion, tender watercress and a drink from the limpid well of Tolain, my need is served and I shall not want.'

WOODRUFF (G. *lus na caithimh*; L. *Asperula odorata*)

The Gaelic name means 'wasting-wort' and the plant was used for treating consumption and other cheat troubles.

WOOD SORREL (G. *seamrag*; L. *Oxalis acetosella*)

The Revd. Angus MacFarlane described the wood sorrel thus:

> It is a dainty little thing; and the whole plant a perfect hydroscope, the delicate trifoliate leaf folding into a triangular pyramid, and the exquisitely veined, lilac-coloured corolla closing up before rain or whenever the sun goes down. It grows in sheltered situations in wood and under bushes, being copious in its habits. Children like to munch the leaves, which have a very agreeable acid taste, grateful on a hot day. As the leaves, however, are very small, it was usual to gather a goodly bunch to make it worthwhile and get the full benefit. This we called Greim saighdeir, a soldier's mouthful. I suppose it would take many such mouthfuls to produce the minimum of salts of sorrel that would be fatal. Yet we were often warned that eating too generously of the leaves had been known to be followed by ill-effects. But little heed will childen give to such; witness their habit of sucking the honey-bags of the foxglove flowers. Wonderful is their immunity. [33]

It was boiled in water and the resulting liquid quenched the thirst and lowered the temperatures of feverish patients. In Arran a whey or tea of it was used in 'putrid fever' (typhus) with, it was claimed, 'good success'.

WORMWOOD (G. *burmaid*; L. *Artemesia absinthium*)

Wormwood was collected in September before the frost came, when the fruit would be ripe and the stem and leaves nearly dry. It was kept by hanging it from the ceiling in a muslin bag, and when needed an infusion was made of about two ounces of dried herb to one pint of boiling water. It was used as a vermifuge with considerable success. One teaspoonful was a dose for children and adults were given a maximum of a tablespoonful.

YARROW (G. *Earr-thalmhainn* or *Lus chasgadh na fala*; L. *Achillea millifolium*)

The yarrow was a potent styptic. John Lightfoot wrote in 1777:

> The highlanders still continue to make an ointment of it to heal and dry
> up wounds. The common people, in order to cure the headache, do
> sometimes thrust a leaf of it up their nostrils to make their nose bleed. [34]

It was also a lovers' herb. Young girls would cut it before sunrise,
place it under their pillow and hope to dream of their sweetheart. If
his back was turned towards them in the dream it meant that they
would never marry. If he faced them, marriage would surely follow.

And the Last Word in Cures . . .

If everything else failed, the Gaelic healers had an awesome panacea.
The following charm was said to be a cure for all the ills that flesh
is heir to:

> Ola cas easgainn,
> Bainne-cìch circe,
> Is geir mheanbhchuileag
> Ann an adharc muice,
> Agus ite cait ga shuathadh ris.
> Oil from an eel's foot,
> Milk from a hen's teat,
> And the tallow of midges
> [Blended] In the horn of a pig,
> And rubbed on with a feather from a cat's wing. [1]

There is wisdom as well as drollery in that, if we think about it.

NOTES ON SOURCES

INTRODUCTION: Ambiguities of Art and Healing

1   For a general perspective on Celtic art and design from the Iron Age to the late
    medieval West Highland monuments and the nineteenth century revival, see
    Laing, Lloyd and Jennifer, *Art of the Celts*, Thames & Hudson, London, 1992.
2   McCutcheon, Alexander, 'Some Highland Household Remedies', *Pharmaceu-
    tical Journal & Pharmacist*, 19 April, 1919, 235–6.
3   Foskett, R., *The Zambesi Journals of Dr John Kirk*, Appendix 1, Edinburgh, 1965.
4   Ross, Andrew, 'The Scottish Missionary Doctor' in Derek A. Dow (ed.)
    The Influence of Scottish Medicine, Parthenon Publishing Group, Carnforth,
    Lancashire and New Jersey, 1988, 95.
5   Cooper, Derek, *Road to the Isles: Travellers in the Hebrides 1770–1914*, Richard
    Drew, Glasgow, 1990, is a perceptive account, with lengthy extracts, of
    visitors' views of Scottish Gaeldom.
6   Jenkinson, Jacqueline, *Scottish Medical Societies 1731–1939: Their History and
    Records*, Edinburgh University Press, writes:

> The Caledonian Medical Society was first established as a student society
> by a small group of Highland medical students at the University of
> Edinburgh, which met briefly between February and April in 1878. The
> official date of formation is given in the Society's *Medical Directory* entries
> as 1881, when the Society was reconvened and its rules revised. The
> intention of the originators of the Society to promote the study of Celtic
> folk-medicine, ancient and contemporary, was continued as the Society
> expanded . . . [Membership was] open to University medical graduates of
> Highland descent. The Society had 20 members in 1885, and 36 in 1889.
> By 1906, the total membership was 232.

It published the *Caledonian Medical Journal* between 1883 and 1968.
7   Black, R., *Catalogue of Classical Gaelic Manuscripts. in the National Library of
    Scotland*, forthcoming.

8 Shaw, Francis, 'Irish Medical Men and Philosophers', in Brian O Cuív (ed.), *Seven Centuries of Irish Learning*, Dublin, 1961.

I HISTORY

1 Origins

1 Quoted in Thomson, Derick, *An Introduction to Gaelic Poetry*, Victor Gollancz, London, 1974, 148.

2 For a discussion of the symbolism of the caduceus see Hall, James, *Dictionary of Subjects and Symbols in Art*, John Murray, London, rev. edn, 1979; and Circlot, J. E., *A Dictionary of Symbols*, trans. Jack Sage, Routledge & Kegan Paul, London 1962.

3 The old spelling of 'Rum' is used for the island as it is now coming back into use, having been formally re-adopted by its present owners, Scottish Natural Heritage. 'Rhum' was largely a nineteenth-century invention.

4 The full record of the Rum excavations is given in Wickham-Jones, Caroline, *Rhum: Mesolithic and Later Sites at Kinloch: Excavations 1984–86*, Society of Antiquaries of Scotland, Monograph Series No 7, Edinburgh, 1990.

5 Sisson, C. H., *In a Trojan Ditch*, Carcanet Press, Manchester, 1974.

6 The goddess and the saint are referred to as Brigid and St Brigid respectively, to avoid confusion with other forms such as Bride, Brìghd, and the Gaelic genitive, Brìghde. Similarly, readily recognised forms of other names are used.

2 Magical Water and Smelly Onions

1 Cowie, Trevor G., *Magic Metal: Early Metalworkers in the North-East*, Anthropological Museum, University of Aberdeen, 1988, gives a concise and authoritative account of the importance of metal and water in Bronze Age rituals.

2 For a splendid introduction to Celtic literature see Jackson, Kenneth, *A Celtic Miscellany*, Routledge & Kegan Paul, London, 1951 (rev. edn, Penguin Books, 1971). The preliminary note to the section on 'Nature' is particularly relevant here.

3 'Such projects would have involved huge expenditure of human energy: estimates range from 80,000 man hours for the construction of the henge at Ring of Brogar, Orkney to around 3,500,000 for the great passage grave at Newgrange in the Boyne Valley, Ireland.' Cowie, op. cit.

4 Glob, P. V., *The Mound People: Danish Bronze-Age Man Preserved*, Faber & Faber, London, 1974, 162.

5 Sutherland, Revd. G., *Folklore Gleanings and Character Sketches from the Far North*, John o'Groat Journal, Wick, 1937,63–7.

6 Glob, op. cit., 162.

7 Chamberlain, Mary, *Old Wives' Tales: Their History, Remedies and Spells*, Virago, London, 1981, 5.

8 Tacitus, *Germania*, in *The Agricola and the Germania*, trans. H. Mattingly & S. A. Handford, Penguin Books, London, 1988.

Notes On Sources

9   Tacitus, *Annals of Imperial Rome*, trans. Michael Grant, Cassell, London, 1963.
10 Ross, Anne, *Pagan Celtic Britain*, Routledge & Kegan Paul, London, 1967 and Sphere Books, 1974, 316.
11 Piggott, Stuart, *The Druids*, Thames & Hudson, London, 1968, and Penguin Books, 1978, 108.
12 In Gaelic mythology the *Tuatha Dé Danaan*, People of the Goddess Danu, were semi-divine and divine beings who inhabited Ireland before the Celts and Gaels.
13 There was an unfortunate side-effect to this 'cure'. Ever afterwards the poor doorkeeper's cat's eye stayed awake all night looking for mice.
14 The first known mention of the Picts as such is by the Roman writer Eumenius in AD 297, but it is generally accepted that the Caledonii referred to by Tacitus in his *Agricola* were a Pictish tribe. Modern archaeology tends to the belief that these people were the descendants of the Bronze Age – if not earlier – natives of northern Scotland. It is also possible that Pictish culture, as it is understood today, was introduced by an incoming, dominant warrior aristocracy, while the aboriginal population, already long permeated by and interbred with the descendants of Neolithic farmers and other immigrants, adopted, by gentle or forceful persuasion, new ways alongside their older traditions. Despite the aura of mystery that continues to surround them, the Picts are, in many ways, the most thoroughly investigated of all the north-west European Iron Age peoples. It is known that they were skilled builders, farmers and traders, and that they patronised gifted artists in sculpture and metalwork. At a time when most of Europe and the rest of the British Isles were involved in tremendous social upheavals and wars, the Picts appear to have retained a notably stable society despite their own troubles with invading forces. What is lacking is their own written records, and historians have had to rely on the accounts of Romans, Anglians – such as Bede – and the incoming Gaels of Ireland, with all of whom they were in conflict, and none of whom therefore can be guaranteed as unbiased.
15 Ross, Anne, *Everyday Life of the Pagan Celts*, Batsford, London, 1970, 108.
16 Brønsted, Johannes, *The Vikings*, trans. Kalle Skov, Penguin Books, Harmondsworth, 1965, 254.

3 Monks and Medicine
1 The form Calum Cille is used throughout for St Columba.
2 Anderson, A. O. and M. O., (eds & trans), *Adomnán's Life of Columba*, Clarendon Press, Oxford, 1991, 147.
3 Anderson, op. cit., 143.
4 Cowan, Ian B. and Easson, David E., *Medieval Religious Houses: Scotland*, Longman, London, 2nd edn, 1976, 162–200.

4 Clan Patronage and Medieval Medicine
1 MacBeth itself was an early medieval Gaelic forename meaning 'Son of Life', but the obvious clumsiness of developing its correct form as Mac-MacBeth soon led to the dropping of one of the 'macs'. The Beaton form probably came

about through the scotticising of the scholarly Latin style of the name, Betonus, increasingly adopted, after the medieval fashion, by those Highland doctors who studied in Continental universities and medical schools. Another influence in the scotticising of the name may have come from supposed connections with the Bethune/Beatons of Fife, an established Lowland family (of which Cardinal David Beaton (1494–1546) was a member), with thirteenth-century origins in Béthune, in French Flanders. In later times spellings of the Macbeth lineage vary from MacVeagh and MacVey to Bethune and Paton.

2   John Bannerman's *The Beatons: A Medical Kindred in the Classical Gaelic Tradition*, John Donald, Edinburgh, 1986, is the outcome of fine scholarship and wide-ranging research and gives a wealth of information on the genealogies, landholdings and education of the medieval Beaton doctors. This chapter concentrates more on the medicines and folklore memories of the doctors on which Bannerman barely touches. Many lengthy conversations with Ronald Black have been invaluable in providing information on the subject, and he has also provided a great deal of information by way of written communications.

3   Nicholson, A., 'The McBeths: hereditary physicians of the Highlands', in *Transactions of the Gaelic Society of Glasgow*, vol. 5, Glasgow, 1958.

4   Thomson, Derick, 'Gaelic Learned Orders and Literati in Medieval Scotland', in *Scottish Studies*, vol. 12, part 1, Edinburgh, 1968.

5   Bannerman, op. cit., 82.

6   Quoted in Henderson, George, *The Norse Influence on Celtic Scotland*, Glasgow, 1910.

7   *Dates and Documents relating to the Family and Property of Sutherland extracted chiefly from the Originals in the Charter Room at Dunrobin*, compiled by the then Sutherland Estates factor, James Loch, in 1859. Copies of the charters are in the Reay Papers (GD84) and the originals (RH6 1/74 and RH6 1/86) are in Register House, Edinburgh. My thanks to Olive Geddes of the National Library of Scotland for tracing the whereabouts of these charters.

8   A note to a record of the documents held by the House of Sutherland, James Loch, op. cit., refers to the process by which the island's name was changed.

9   Similar reasons have been put forward for sixteenth-century Ireland by Professor Brian O Cuív in Moody, Martin, Byrne (eds), *A New History of Ireland*, vol. III, Oxford, 1976, 518:

> One important factor in this survival is that members of medical families were given to compiling books for their own use and for fellow doctors, and that such books were commonly retained within the family circle of the owner. An indication of the value placed on such manuscripts is the fact that in 1500 the Earl of Kildare gave twenty cows for the manuscript of a medical textbook. There is also the fact that Irish medical men do not seem to have been subjected to the same criticism and harsh treatment as members of the other hereditary professions, possibly because their services were useful to members of the English colony, and also because of the European element in their educational background which they shared

with English and continental doctors. Hence in the sixteenth century we find Irish leeches active throughout the four provinces and even practising in Dublin.

Ronald Black has noted: 'All of Ò Cuív's points hold good for Scotland.'

10 From a note in Donald Macqueen's hand accompanying his gift of Farquhar Beaton of Husabost's copy of Bernard Gordon's *Lilium Medicinae* to the Society of Antiquaries of Scotland in 1784. Recorded in Mackinnon, D., *A Descriptive Catalogue of Gaelic Manuscripts in the Advocates' Library, Edinburgh, and elsewhere in Scotland*, 1912, 298.

11 Collins, Kenneth, *Go and Learn: the international story of Jews and Medicine in Scotland*, Aberdeen University Press, Aberdeen, 1988, 3. Of the interaction between Jewish, Arabian and European medicine in the Middle Ages, Collins remarks on the same page 'The role of the Jewish physician as translator should not be underestimated for Arabic and Greek medical works could be translated into Latin and Hebrew, and vice versa. Thus Jewish physicians helped to transmit Greek medicine to the Arab world and Arab medicine to Europe.' As his name tells us, the philosopher-physician Isaac was from Israel but he spent his early life in North Africa and wrote in Arabic.

12 Advocates' MS 72.1.2, translation supplied by Ronald Black.

13 Macdonald, Joan, *An Edition of a Gaelic Medical Manuscript*, unpublished MA dissertation, University of Edinburgh, 1991. Her translation and notes on lengthy extracts from Advocate's Manuscript 72.2.10 (National Library of Scotland) have been indispensable in gaining an insight into the workings of the Beaton doctors' medical practice and a deeper knowledge of their materia medica.

14 Mackechnie, John, (ed.), *The Dewar Manuscripts*, vol. 1, Maclellan, Glasgow, 1963, 367 n. 566.

15 Letters on Customs and Antiquities of the Isle of Skye, 1822–3, National Library of Scotland MS 874 ff xxvi, 275–6. Letter to I. Train, Supervision of Excise, South Queensferry, Edinburgh, from John Kelly, in Dunvegan.

16 Maclean, Norman, *The Former Days*, Hodder & Stoughton, London, 1945, 34.

17 Helen Lindsay, *Folklore of Dunbeath*, Dunbeath Preservation Trust, 1985.

18 This Kilpheadar, in the north-west of North Uist, is now deserted and part of the farm of Balelone and is not to be confused with the still viable South Uist township of the same name. I am indebted to Joan Troughton of Carinish, North Uist, for enlightening me on this point.

19 The information on the Dotair Bàn and his family is from Norman Macdonald's booklet *Trinity Temple, Carinish, North Uist*, and from Dr M.D. Macleod's memoir of his grandfather in the *Caledonian Medical Journal*, vol. II, no. 8. I am also grateful for information from Dr Sorley MacLean. Further details on the Macleods of Rigg and Raasay may be found in A. Morrison's *Genealogy of Lewis and Raasay*, vol. 2.

20 Macleod, M.D., op. cit.

21 Sources for information on the medical men of the Forty-Five are given in the Select Bibliography.

5 Highland Medicine and the Enlightenment

1 Ferguson, William, *Scotland: 1689 to the Present*, vol IV of *The Edinburgh History of Scotland*, Oliver & Boyd, Edinburgh and London, 1968, 209.

2 Martin, M., *A Description of the Western Islands of Scotland*, London, 2nd edn, 1716 (facsimile, James Thin, 1976), x–xi.

3 Martin, 1716, op. cit., xi–xii.

4 Martin, 1716, op. cit., xii–xiii.

5 Martin, M., *A Voyage to St Kilda*, 4th edn, London, 1753, 40.

6 Martin, 1753, op. cit., 40–1.

7 Carmichael, Alexander, *Carmina Gadelica: Hymns and incantations*, 6. vols., Edinburgh, 1900–71. He discusses *Eòlas nan Neòn*, the Charm of the Styes, in volume 4, 218–9. With the exception of the story of the *ballan* in Chapter 12, all the other *Carmina* references given here are for the English-only version, Floris Books, Edinburgh, 1992.

8 Carmichael, op. cit., Floris, 1992, 646–7. The verses of the incantation are quoted on page 396.

6 Folk Healers

1 Larner, Christina, Lee, Christopher Hyde, & McLachlan, Hugh V., *A Source-Book of Scottish Witchcraft*, Glasgow, 1977.

2 Dalyell, John Graham, *The Darker Superstitions of Scotland*, Glasgow, 1835, 27.

3 Trial of Agnes Sampsoun, Nether Keith, 1590. Justiciary Court MS 26/2 (Scottish Record Office). The prayers referred to are quoted in John Graham Dalyell, op. cit., 24–6.

4 For example, J. G. Campbell, George Sutherland, Alexander Stewart ('Nether Lochaber').

5 The case is recounted in J. G. Dalyell, op. cit., 170–5. An account of the trial occurs in R. Pitcairn, *Criminal Trials in Scotland*, VI, part 2, Edinburgh, 1833.

6 Dalyell, op. cit., 172.

7 Laurence Gomme's 'Ethnology in Folklore' (London 1892), notes nineteenth-century instances of sacrifices of cattle not only in Ireland & Scotland, but also in Wales, Yorkshire, Northamptonshire, Cornwall and the Isle of Man. 'Within twenty miles of the metropolis of Scotland a relative of Professor Simpson offered up a live cow as a sacrifice to the spirit of the murrain.' Such a practice may owe not a little to 19th century antiquarian revivalism but the same cannot be said for other rural practices which appear to be a direct continuation of a very ancient belief. Charles Squire, *Celtic Myth and Legend* (London, 1905) notes that in Wales it was still customary in the 19th century to throw a bull to its death from a high rock in order to 'cure' various forms of sickness in a herd. In 1859 a Manx farmer offered a heifer as a burnt offering near Tynwald Hill, to avert the anger of the ghostly occupant of a burial mound which had been disturbed. Sometimes, as in the Loch Maree cases, these oblations were offered to an alleged Christian saint. In Kirkcudbright, St Cuthbert, and at Clynnog, Wales, St Beuno, were thought to delight in the blood of bulls.

8   Macleod of Macleod, R. C., *The Book of Dunvegan*, vol. 1 (1340–1700), Aberdeen, 1888.

9   Martin, 1716, op. cit., 197–9.

10 Fraser, H. E., 'Some Notes on the Popular Medicine and Surgery of the Highlands of Scotland', *Caledonian Medical Journal*, vol. II, 1886, 265. The Gaelic spelling has been amended.

11 Logan, J. R., 'Popular Medicine and Surgery of the Highlands of Scotland', in *Caledonian Medical Journal*, vol. II, 1896, 279–80.

12 The connotations of the English term 'witch', the usual translation of *buisdeach*, make for an uneasy image in the context of Gaelic traditions. Readers are referred to the introduction to J. G. Campbell's *Witchcraft in the Scottish Highlands*, in which he discusses the problem.

13 James Robertson's original manuscript, in the Museum of Antiquities' Library, remains unpublished but lengthy extracts and a discussion of the text are in Sir Arthur Mitchell's 'James Robertson's Tour through some of the Western Islands, etc, of Scotland in 1768', *PSAS*, vol. 32, 1897–8.

14 Logan, J. R., op. cit., 282.

15 Masson, D., *Transactions of the Gaelic Society of Inverness (TGSI)*, vol. 14, 1887, 298–313.

16 Grant, Katherine Whyte, 'Old Highland Therapy', in *Caledonian Medical Journal*, Jan. 1904, 365.

17 Martin, 1716, op. cit., 183.

18 Dr Finlay Macleod tells me he thinks the healer in question (unnamed in Henderson's book) was probably a Norman Macdonald of Cross in north Lewis, a notable healer.

19 Henderson, George, 1910, op. cit., 319–320.

20 Logan, J. R., op. cit., 281–2.

21 Macgregor, Alastair, 'Popular Medicine and Surgery of the Highlands of Scotland', *Caledonian Medical Journal*, vol. II, 286.

7   Lairds, Ministers and Dominies

1   Thomson, Derick, *An Introduction to Gaelic Poetry*, op. cit., 223.

2   Macgregor, Duncan, 'Old Highland Remedies', *Caledonian Medical Journal*, vol. II, 1896, 278–9.

3   Sage, Revd. Donald, *Memorabilia Domestica: or Parish Life in the North of Scotland*, 2nd edn, William Rae, Wick, and John Menzies, Edinburgh, 1899, 133.

8   'As Long as Grass Grows'

1   The Society was formed in Inverness in 1817 and continued until 1829. Its objects, according to the *Inverness Journal* for 9 May 1817, were 'promoting Medical Science, and establishing a Professional Library'.

2   *Rules adopted by the Medical Society of the North for the Regulation of their Fees*, Inverness, 1818.

3   *Old Statistical Account for Caithness and Sutherland*. The OSAs were published in Edinburgh, 1790–8.

4 The story is meticulously recounted in local oral tradition to this day.

5 There are a several books which detail the excesses of the Clearances, their aftermath, and the struggle to regain security of land tenure. They are listed under Select Bibliography. It has been argued by some, in particular Rosalind Mitchison ('The Highland Clearances' *Scottish Economic and Social History*, vol. 1, no. 1, 1981), that 'the whole subject is heavy with myth' and that much of the evidence, taken down much later, at the time of the Napier Commission investigations in the 1880s, was unreliable and biased. Professor Mitchison reproves her fellow historian, Dr William Ferguson, for using the word 'brutally' in describing the Strathnaver evictions, 'as if the use of physical force had been established'. She may justifiably argue, as others have done, that the impassioned testimony of some, such as the Strathnaver stonemason Donald Macleod, in *Gloomy Memories*, is emotionally overcharged (and in the circumstances, understandably so), but other first-hand accounts, such as that of the Revd. Donald Sage, the minister of the mission at Achness, Strathnaver, may be taken as more objective. Despite concern for his flock, Sage was curiously away at his father's house in the Strath of Kildonan at the height of the evictions, but of his journey through Strathnaver in the following week he remarked:

> The spectacle present was hideous and ghastly! The banks of the lake and the river, formerly studded with cottages, now met the eye as a scene of desolation. Of all the houses, the thatched roofs were gone, but the walls, built of alternate layers of turf and stone, remained. The flames of the preceding week still slumbered in their ruins, and sent up into the air spiral columns of smoke; whilst here a gable, and there a long side-wall, undermined by the fire burning within them, might be seen tumbling to the ground, from which a cloud of smoke, and then a dusky flame, slowly sprang up. The sooty rafters of the cottages, as they were being consumed, filled the air with a heavy and most offensive odour.

Sage's private journal, edited by his son and published posthumously in 1889 as *Memorabilia Domestica*, is worth reading not only for its account of the Strathnaver Clearance, but also for its wide-ranging information on Highland life of the period.

6 The eruption of Laki Giga in Iceland in 1783 compounded the effect of the little Ice Age which lasted from about 1650 to 1850. The clouds of poisonous dust and gases it created, at the time described as 'noxious dews', led to blackened and scorched grassland and leaf-drop from trees throughout a wide area of Europe. Thus natural disaster played its part in the discontent that led to the French Revolution of 1789–97.

7 As Marquis of Stafford, the first Duke of Sutherland had been appointed British Ambassador to France in 1790. In August 1792 when the mob stormed the royal palace, killed the guards and imprisoned Louis XVI and Marie Antoinette in the Temple, the Countess of Sutherland (Marchioness of Stafford) befriended the queen and arranged for clothes and linen to be smuggled into the prison for

her use. Six weeks later the Ambassador and his wife and children were safely returned to Britain. (See *Looking Back: The Autobiography of the* [fifth] *Duke of Sutherland*, Odhams, London, 1957.)

Thomas Paine's *The Rights of Man*, 1791, which defended the French Revolution, sold well in Scotland – where sympathy for the republican cause was stronger than in England – and was the subject of a popular verse:

> The Rights of Man is now well kenned
> And read by mony a hunder
> For Tammy Paine the buik has penned
> And lent the court a lounder.
>
> (*Lounder*: a hefty knock)

8 Grant, Katherine Whyte, op. cit., 369–70.

9 Quoted in Temperley, Alan, *Tales of the North Coast*, Research Publishing Company, London, 1977, 245–6.

10 Dewar Report: *Report of the Committee on the Highlands and Islands Medical Services*, HMSO, 1912.

11 Scottish Home & Health Dept, *General Medical Services in the Highlands & Islands*, HMSO, Edinburgh, 1967.

9 A Future for the Past?

1 Akerele, Olayiwola, 'Which way for traditional medicine', *World Health*, magazine of the World Health Organisation, Geneva, June 1983. At the time of writing Dr Akerele was director of the Traditional Medicine unit at the WHO headquarters in Geneva.

2 Eliot, George, *Silas Marner: The Weaver of Raveloe* (1861), Penguin Books, 1967, 200.

II MATERIA MEDICA

10 Water, Wells and Healing Springs

1 W. J. Watson, *The History of the Celtic Placenames of Scotland* (1926; repr. Irish Academic Press, 1973) is an authoritative treasure house of information. W. F. H. Nicolaisen, *Scottish Place-names*, is a natural follow-up to Watson's seminal work and takes a close look at underlying trends in Scottish place-names.

1 Anderson, op. cit., 109–11.

3 James M. Mackinlay, *Folklore of Scottish Lochs and Springs* (Glasgow, 1893). I am also indebted to the records of the Royal Commission on the Ancient & Historical Monuments of Scotland.

4 There is a sizeable Scottish contribution on these sites in *Burnt Offerings* (Wordwell Academic Publications, Dublin, 1990) compiled by Victor Buckley from papers read at the first international conference on burnt mounds held in Dublin in 1988.

5 Martin, 1716, op. cit., 189.

6 Pennant, Thomas, *A Tour in Scotland and Voyage to the Hebrides*, 1772. Quoted in

James M. Mackinlay's *Folklore of Scottish Lochs and Springs*, Glasgow, 1893, 29.

7   Macphail, S. Rutherford, 'Notes on Highland Charms and Worshipping of Holy Wells', *Caledonian Medical Journal*, vol. II, 1896, 271.

8   Macgregor, Duncan, op. cit., 274.

9   MacPhail, op. cit., 272.

10 Martin, 1753, op. cit., 16.

11 Grant, Katherine Whyte, op. cit., 361.

11   The Enchantment of Stone and Metal

1   Quoted in Mircea Eliade's *History of Religious Ideas*, vol. I, *From the Stone Age to the Eleusinian Mysteries*, Collins, London, 1979, 115.

2   Hugh Miller, *The Old Red Sandstone*, Edinburgh, 1841, quoted in George Rosie's *Hugh Miller: Outrage and Order*, Mainstream, Edinburgh, 1981, 196.

3   Miller, 1841, quoted in Rosie, op. cit., 197.

4   Macdonald, Revd. Norman, 'Notes on Gaelic Folklore II', in *Arv: Tidskrift för Nordisk Folkminnesforskning: Journal of Scandinavian Folklore*, vol. 17, 1961, Uppsala & Copenhagen, 197.

5   Fraser, H. E., 'Some Notes on the Popular Medicine and Surgery of the Highlands of Scotland', *Caledonian Medical Journal*, vol. II, 1886, 262–3.

6   Green, Miranda J., *Dictionary of Celtic Myth and Legend*, Thames & Hudson, London, 1992.

7   *PSAS*, vol. 13, 107.

8   Quoted in Black, George F, 'Scottish Charms and Amulets', *PSAS*, vol. 27, 1892–3, 520.

9   Ritchie, Anna, 'Painted pebbles in early Scotland', *PSAS*, vol. 104, Edinburgh, 1971–2, 299.

10 Ritchie, op. cit., 299.

11 Thomas Davidson, 'Animal Treatment in Eighteenth-Century Scotland', *Scottish Studies*, vol. 4.

12 Sutherland, Revd. George, op. cit., 126–7.

13 Black, George F., 'Scottish Charms and Amulets', in *PSAS*, vol. 27, 1892–3, 433–526. An invaluable source of information on healing stones and other talismans.

14 Paton, Sir Noel, in *PSAS* vol. xxi, 228.

15 Royalty and the aristocracy, perhaps being less prone to having self-confidence in old traditions undermined because their status itself was enshrined and validated by custom, often shared with the peasantry archaic practices from which the middle-classes were increasingly to shy away. In the fifteenth and sixteenth centuries, for example, the queens of Scotland wore the 'Sanct Margaretis sark', a garment belonging to Margaret, wife of Malcolm Canmore, when in labour. They believed that this would lessen their pains. Less well-connected Lowland women had to be content with invoking the saintly queen, as Sir David Lindsay (1486–1555) wrote:

> Sum wyffis Sanct Margaret doith exhort,
> Into thair birth thame to support.

16   Black, George, op. cit., 441.

17   Stokes, Whitley, (ed.), *Lives of Saints from the Book of Lismore*, Clarendon Press, Oxford, 1890, 288. My thanks to John Purser for drawing my attention to the use of bells in healing.

18   Fraser, H. E., op. cit., 263.

19   Macdonald, Revd. James, *TGSI*, vol. xix, 274.

12   Of Mice, Horns and Butterflies

1   There are discussions of these prescriptions in D. L.Cowen 'The Edinburgh Pharmacopoeia' *Medical History*, vol. 1, 1957; and in C. G. Drummond, 'Pharmacy and medicine in Old and New Edinburgh', *Scottish Genealogist, vol.* 12, no. i, 1965.

2   Carmichael, *Carmina Gadelica*, vol. 4, 1941, 205.

3   Macphail, op. cit., 270.

4   Marwick, Ernest, *The Folklore of Orkney and Shetland*, Batsford, London, 1975, 130.

5   Martin, 1716, op. cit., 146.

6   Bryce, Derek, (ed.) *The Herbal Remedies of the Physicians of Myddfai*, trans. John Pugh, Llanerch, Lampeter, 1987, 45.

7   Mackenzie, Donald A., 'Oriental Elements in Scottish Mythology', in *TGSI*, 1922. Mackenzie gives no published source for his quotations from Professor Elliot Smith and Dr Netolitzsky.

8   But in *Story and Song from Loch Ness-side*, Alexander Macdonald writes, 'A tooth broken or extracted should be thrown into the fire; if the mice got it, no new tooth would grow, and so much of the person's entirety was gone.'

9   Quoted in Campbell, J. L., and Thomson, Derick, *Edward Lhuyd in the Scottish Highlands 1699–1700*, Clarendon, Oxford, 1963, 63–4.

10   Fraser, H. E., op. cit., 260.

11   Matheson, Neil, 'Highland Healers', *Scots Magazine*, Feb. 1949, 391.

12   Grant, Katherine Whyte, op. cit., 370–1.

13   Rituals, Charms and Incantations

1   William Mackenzie's paper 'Gaelic Incantations' is in the *Transactions of the Gaelic Society of Inverness*, vol. 18, 189–2. Other sources are John Gregorson Campbell's *Witchcraft and Second Sight in the Highlands*, 1902; Alexander Macdonald's *Story and Song from Loch Ness-side*, 1914, and the same author's 'Medical Spells and Charms of the Highlands' in the *Celtic Magazine*, vol. 13, 1887–8, as well as Alexander Carmichael's *Carmina Gadelica*. A sympathetic modern view of the efficacy of charms is that of Dr Patrick Logan, who writes in *Making the Cure* (Dublin, 1972):

> Even today the best medicine is reassurance and the ability to reassure a patient does not always go with a medical degree . . . It is likely that the use of a charm with its air of mystery and hidden power would be more effective, in the case of some patients, than an official remedy . . . Almost all physical illnesses – over 80% of them – will get better no matter

what treatment is given, so it is only common sense on the part of the medical attendant to make sure that he will be given the credit for the favourable result.

2   Quoted in Mackenzie, Wm, op. cit., 98–9.

3   *Conair* and *connachair* remain untranslated in the published versions of this incantation known to me. However, Dwelly's *Dictionary* gives several meanings for *conair*: Way, course, path or circle. Perhaps some 'path' or 'circle' was drawn by the person transmitting the Evil Eye. A *conachair* is a sick person who gets neither worse or better, and Dwelly refers the reader to *conghair*: uproar, clamour, confusion, tumult, fury.

4   Mackenzie, Wm, op cit., 135–6.

5   Mackenzie, Wm, op. cit., 134.

6   Mackenzie, Wm, op. cit., 113–4.

7   Stokes, Whitley & Strachan, John, (eds), *Thesaurus Palaeohibernicus*, vol. 2, Cambridge University Press, 1903, 248–9. In the versions quoted here Ronald Black has kindly provided modernised versions of the rather dated translations of the St Gall incantations by Stokes and Strachan.

8   Stokes & Strachan, op. cit.

9   Stokes & Strachan, op. cit.

10 Stokes & Strachan, op. cit.

11 Mackenzie, Wm, op. cit., 168.

12 Logan, Patrick, *Making the Cure: A Look at Irish Folk Medicine*, Talbot Press, Dublin, 1972, 62.

13 Sutherland, Revd. George, op. cit., 108.

14 Mackenzie, Wm, op. cit., 138–9.

15 I have been asked to preserve both the anonymity of my informants and the name of the island in question. However, Margaret Mackay of Edinburgh University has recorded the ritual and its accompanying incantation in words and photographs for the archives of the School of Scottish Studies. Sensitive information held by the School is released only after an agreed number of years, which may be several decades.

14   Herbal

1   Adv. MS. 72.1.2, National Library of Scotland; trans Ronald Black.

2   Martin, 1716, op. cit., 41.

3   Charles Alston's *Lectures in Materia Medica*, 2 vols., Edinburgh, 1776, makes the argument plain. Alston was the first professor of botany at Edinburgh, and his lively lectures, collected and published by his students after his death, are very useful for checking medical and botanical terminology of the period, since he gives a variety of alternative terms in use during his own and previous times.

4   An article by the author in the *West Highland Free Press* (9 Oct. 1992) looks more fully into the confusion over the germander speedwell though it contains an error in saying that the plant is not mentioned in Cameron's *Gaelic Names of Plants* – it is given in the amended second edition.

Notes On Sources

5   Lightfoot, Revd. John, *Flora Scotica*, 2 vols., London, 1777, vol. 1, 201.

6   MacFarlane, Revd. Angus, 'Gaelic Names of Plants: study of their uses and lore', *TGSI*, vol. 32, 1922–24, 21.

7   Fairweather, Barbara, *Highland Plant Lore*, Glencoe & North Lorn Folk Museum, undated, but *c*.1975. The pages in this small but useful booklet are unnumbered but the method of making bogbean tonic is given among the plants listed for the month of May.

8   Maclean, Alistair, *Hebridean Altars: Some Studies of the Spirit of an Island Race*, Moray Press, Edinburgh & London, 1937, 21.

9   MacFarlane, op. cit., 23.

10 Pennant, 1769 edn, op. cit., vol. III, 42.

11 Macdonald, Revd. Norman, op. cit., 193.

12 McCutcheon, Alexander, 'Some Highland Household Remedies', *Pharmaceutical Journal and Pharmacist*, 19 April, 1919, 235.

13 Lightfoot, op. cit., vol. 2, 1078.

14 The note, undated, is in the handwriting of Isabel Grant who founded the Highland Folk Museum at Kingussie in 1944. After a lifetime devoted to Scottish history and culture (especially what she called 'the homely, ancient Highland things') Dr Grant died in 1983 at the age of ninety-six.

15 Ann MacDonell, pers. comm.

16 See n. 4 above.

17 Buchanan, George, Rerum Scoticarum Historia (1582), trans. James Aikman, *The History of Scotland, trans. from the Latin of George Buchanan*, 4 vols., Glasgow, 1827. The quotation here is from *Monro's Western Isles of Scotland* (1549), edited by R. W. Munro, Oliver & Boyd, Edinburgh & London, 1961, 43.

18 McCutcheon, op. cit., 235

19 McCutcheon, op. cit., 235

20 Lightfoot, op. cit., vol. 2, 621.

21 Macgregor, Duncan, op. cit., 277.

22 McCutcheon, op. cit., 235

23 Macgregor, Duncan, op. cit., 277–8.

24 Macdonald, Revd. Norman, op. cit., 193.

25 Macgregor, Alastair, op. cit., 287.

26 Martin, 1716, op. cit., 148.

27 Macgregor, Duncan, op. cit., 277.

28 Macphail, Rutherford, op. cit., 270.

29 MacFarlane, op. cit., 12–3.

30 Lightfoot, op. cit., vol. 1., 389–90.

31 Pennant, 1769 edn, op. cit., vol. III, 43.

32 Martin, op. cit., 179–80.

33 MacFarlane, op. cit., 11.

34 Lightfoot, op. cit., vol. 1, 496.

And the Last Word in Cures

1   Mackenzie, Wm, op. cit., 176.

SELECT BIBLIOGRAPHY

The books and journals listed below do not represent all the published sources referred to in the course of researching this work and none of the primary (unpublished) sources, but are chosen largely for the general reader. A selection of rather more academic works is included for those readers who may wish to explore the subject in greater depth. Some of the books given for earlier historical chapters (for example Martin Martin's *A Description of the Western Islands of Scotland*) are also relevant background reading for the cures in Part II – this will be clear from references in the main text. Several small museums and libraries throughout the Highlands and islands have useful information on traditional medicine. The one at Kingussie has a worthwhile documentary archive. The West Highland Museum in Fort William has a number of charm-stones and seed amulets formerly in the private collection of Alexander Carmichael.

GENERAL

Beith, Mary, 'Deanamh a' Leighis: Gaelic Medical Tradition', in *West Highland Free Press*, fortnightly column, 7 July 1989 –

Caledonian Medical Journal, Edinburgh, 1883–1968, especially the early volumes 1890–1910, contain a wealth of papers on Highland folk remedies.

Comrie, J. D., *History of Scottish Medicine*, 2 vols., Wellcome, London, 2nd edn, 1932.

Dwelly, Edward, *Illustrated Gaelic-English Dictionary*, 8th edn. Gairm, Glasgow, 1973. A treasure-trove of Gaelic words and phrases with numerous source references and extended explanations of many terms. Those needing a dictionary with an English-Gaelic section and a guide to pronouncing Gaelic words are referred to Maclennan, Malcolm, below.

Grimble, Ian, *Highland Man*, Highlands & Islands Development Board, Inverness, 1980.

Guthrie, D., *A History of Medicine*, Nelson, London, 1945.

Hamilton, David, *The Healers: A History of Medicine in Scotland*, Canongate, Edinburgh, 1981.

Select Bibliography

Kermack, W. R., *The Scottish Highlands: A Short History*, Johnston & Bacon, Edinburgh & London, 1957.

Larner, Christina, *The Thinking Peasant: Popular and Educated Belief in Pre-Industrial Culture*, Pressgang, Glasgow, 1982.

Logan, Patrick, *Making the Cure: A Look at Irish Folk Medicine*, Talbot Press, Dublin, 1972.

Jackson, K. H., *A Celtic Miscellany*, Routledge & Kegan Paul, London, 1951 (rev. edn, Penguin Books, 1971).

Mackinnon, Charles, *Scottish Highlanders*, Hale, London, 1984.

Maclean, Calum I., *The Highlands*, Batsford, London, 1959. Reprinted: Club Leabhar, Inverness, 1975.

Maclennan, Malcolm, *A Pronouncing and Etymological Dictionary of the Gaelic Language*, Gaelic-English, English-Gaelic, Acair & Aberdeen University Press, reprinted edn 1979.

Masson, D., *TGSI*, vol. 14, 1887, 298–313.

Old Statistical Accounts of Scotland, 1791–8. Parish by parish accounts of contemporary life and local statistics throughout late eighteenth century Scotland, numerous entries on the people's state of health, cures and traditions. Most public libraries stock at least the later bound volumes pertaining to their general area.

Proceedings of the Society of Antiquaries of Scotland. Especially nineteenth-century volumes.

Rhodes, Philip, *An Outline History of Medicine*, Butterworth, London, 1985.

Scottish Home & Health Dept, *General Medical Services in the Highlands & Islands*, HMSO (Cmnd 3257), Edinburgh, 1967, takes a brief but useful look at the history of medicine in the area.

Scottish Studies and *Tocher*, both published regularly by the School of Scottish Studies, Edinburgh, give valuable reports of new research on folklore and social life in Scotland. *Folklore*, the journal of the Folklore Society, also contains Scottish material.

Smout, T. C., *A History of the Scottish People 1560–1830*, Collins, London, 1969.

Thomson, D. S. (ed), *The Companion to Gaelic Scotland*, Blackwell, Oxford, 1983. A new edition was published by Gairm in 1994.

Transactions of the Gaelic Society of Glasgow.

Transactions of the Gaelic Society of Inverness.

West Highland Free Press, Broadford Isle of Skye, 1972 onward. From its inception, the paper has encouraged the publication of features on a broad spectrum of Highland and Island life.

1   Origins

Eliade, Mircea, *History of Religious Ideas*, 3 vols. Collins, London, 1979. Vol. 1, 'From the Stone Age to the Eleusinian Mysteries', throws light on the origins of many later folk practices and theories; chapter 21 of vol. 2, 'From Gautama Buddha to the Triumph of Christianity', sets Celtic religion in a wider context.

Pliny, *Natural History*, 37 books in 10 vols., Loeb Edition, trans. W. H. S. Jones, Harvard University Press, Cambridge, Massachusetts, & Heinemann, London, 1980. Writing in the first century AD, Pliny was fascinated by Celtic customs and it is useful to compare his findings with later Gaelic practices. The work is a mine of information, and Books 20–27 deal with plant products used as medicines; 28–32, medical zoology; and 33–37, minerals (and medicine), the fine arts and gemstones.

Ritchie, J. N. G., & Ritchie, A., *Scotland: Archaeology and Early History*, rev. edn, Edinburgh University Press, 1991.

2 Magical Water and Smelly Onions

Green, Miranda J., *Dictionary of Celtic Myth and Legend*, Thames & Hudson, London, 1992, includes potted backgrounds to a wide variety of deities, places and animals, etc, concerned with healing, accompanied by references for further reading.

Henderson, George, *The Norse Influence on Celtic Scotland*, Glasgow, 1910.

Laing, Lloyd & Jennifer, *Art of the Celts*, Thames & Hudson, London, 1992.

MacCana, Proinsias, *Celtic Mythology*, Hamlyn, London, 1970.

Meldrum, E., ed, *The Dark Ages in the Highlands*, Inverness Field Club, Inverness, 1972.

Ritchie, Anna, *The Kingdom of the Picts*, Chambers, Edinburgh, 1977. Written for schoolchildren, it will be appreciated by adults wanting a clear and authoritative introduction to the subject.

Ross, Anne, *Pagan Celtic Britain*, Routledge & Kegan Paul, London, 1967.
　–*Everyday Life of the Pagan Celts*, Batsford, London, 1970.

Binchy, D. A., 'Bretha Déin Chécht', in *Ériu* vol 19, Dublin, 1962.

Sellar, W. D. H., ed., *Moray: Province and People*, Scottish Society for Northern Studies, Edinburgh, 1993, contains recent research on the Picts.

3 Monks and Medicine

Anderson, A. O. and M. O., (eds & trans), *Adomnàn's Life of Columba*, Clarendon Press, Oxford, 1991.

Cowan, Ian B., and Easson. David E., (eds), *Medieval Religious Houses – Scotland*, Longman, London, 1976 (2nd edn).

Kelly, Fergus, *A Guide to Early Irish Law*, Early Irish Law Series vol. III, Dublin Institute for Advanced Studies, Dublin, 1988.

Moffat, Brian, (ed.) *SHARP Practice: Researches into the Medieval Hospital Soutra*, SHARP, Edinburgh, several volumes, 1986–. Although these are archaeological reports they contain a great deal of information, culled from a variety of sources, on medieval monastic medicine.

4 Clan Patronage and Medieval Medicine

Bannerman, John, *The Beatons: a medical kindred in the classical Gaelic tradition*, John Donald, Edinburgh, 1986.
　–'The Maclachlans of Kilbride and their Manuscripts', in *Scottish Studies*, vol. 21, (1977), 1–34.

Select Bibliography

Best, Richard I., *Bibliography of Irish Philology & Literature*, 2 vols., Dublin 1913 & 1942. Each volume has section on medical works.

Bryce, Derek, ed., *The Herbal Remedies of the Physicians of Myddfai*, Llanerch Enterprises, Lampeter, 1987.

Campbell, Donald, *Arabian Medicine and its Influence on the Middle-Ages*, London, 1926.

Campbell, J. L. and Thompson, D. S. (eds), *Edward Lhuyd in theScottish Highlands 1699–1700*, Oxford, 1963.

Fleetwood, John, *History of Medicine in Ireland*, Dublin, 1951.

Gillies, H. C., *Regimen Sanitatis*, Glasgow, 1911. (Not very reliable but the only Scottish Gaelic medical manuscript in translation which is readily available to the general public via the larger public libraries.)

Grant, I. F., *Highland Folk Ways*, Routledge & Kegan Paul, London & Boston, 1961.

Henslow, G., *Medical Works of the Fourteenth Century*, 1899.

Lloyd, G. E. R., ed., *Hippocratic Writings*, Penguin Books, Harmondsworth, 1978.

Mackay, George, 'Ancient Gaelic Medical Manuscripts', *Caledonian Medical Journal*, vol. 6, 1904.

Mackechnie, John, ed., *The Dewar Manuscripts*, Maclellan, Glasgow, 1963.

Mackechnie, J., *Catalogue of Gaelic Manuscripts in Selected Libraries*, Boston, 1973.

Mackinnon, Donald, *Catalogue of Gaelic Manuscripts in Scotland*, Edinburgh, 1912.

Mackintosh, W. A., 'An Ancient Gaelic Medical Manuscript', *Caledonian Medical Journal*, vol. 7, 1907.

Maclean, Loraine, ed., *The Middle Ages in the Highlands*, Inverness Field Club, Inverness, 1981.

MacNaughton, W. A., *The Medical Heroes of the Forty-Five*, Macdougall, Glasgow, 1867.

Munro, R. W., ed., *Monro's Western Isles of Scotland and Genealogies of the Clans* (1549), Oliver & Boyd, Edinburgh and London, 1961.

Nicholson, A., 'The McBeths – Hereditary Physicians of the Highlands', *Transactions of the Gaelic Society of Glasgow*, vol. 5, 1958.

O'Grady, Standish H., *Catalogue of Irish Manuscripts in the British Museum*, London, 1926.

Shaw, Francis, 'Irish Medical Men & Philosophers' in Brian Ó Cuív, ed., *Seven Centuries of Irish Learning*, Dublin, 1961.

Thomson, Derick, 'Gaelic Learned Orders and Literati in Medieval Scotland', in *Scottish Studies*, vol. 12, Edinburgh, 1968.

Thomson, Derick, *An Introduction to Gaelic Poetry*, Gollancz, London, 1974.

Whittet, Martin M., 'Medical Resources of the Forty-Five', *TGSI*, vol. 44, 1961, 1–40. Whittet's sources are given in full at the end of his paper.

Wulff, W., *Rosa Anglica*, Irish Texts Society, London, 1928.

5   Highland Medicine and the Enlightenment

Alston, Charles, *Lectures in Materia Medica*, Edinburgh, 2 vols, 1776.

Macdonald, C. R., 'St Kilda: its inhabitants and the diseases peculiar to them', *British Medical Journal*, vol. ii, 160, London, 1886.

Martin, Martin, *A Description of the Western Islands of Scotland*, 2nd edn, London, 1716.

Martin, Martin, *A Voyage to St Kilda*, London, 1753.

Underwood, E. A., *Boerhaave's Men at Leyden and After*, Edinburgh, 1977.

Kett, F. P., *The Memoirs of Sir Robert Sibbald: 1641–1722*, London, 1932.

6 Folk Healers

Campbell, John Gregorson, *Witchcraft & Second Sight in the Highlands & Islands of Scotland*, Glasgow, 1902.

Dalyell, J. G., *The Darker Superstitions of Scotland*, Griffin, Glasgow, 1835.

Hand, W. D., 'The folk-healer: calling and endowment', *Journal of the History of Medicine*, vol. 26, 263–275.

Larner, C., *The Enemies of God: The Witch-hunt in Scotland*, Chatto & Windus, London, 1981.

Maclennan, Frank, *Ferindonald Papers*, Ross & Cromarty Heritage Society, Evanton, undated but c.1978. The chapter on Donald Munro, the bonesetter of Knockancuirn, is an excellent study of this category of healer.

McPherson, J. M., *Primitive Beliefs in the North East of Scotland*, Longmans, London, 1929.

Ross, Anne, *The Folklore of the Scottish Highlands*, Batsford, London, 1976.

Sutherland, Revd. George, *Folklore Gleanings and Character Sketches from the Far North*, John O'Groat Journal, Wick, 1937.

7 Lairds, Ministers and Dominies

Brodie, Alexander, *The Diary of Alexander Brodie of Brodie*, Spalding Club, Aberdeen, 1873.

Buchan, William, *Domestic Medicine*, 1769.

Cregeen, Eric, 'The Tacksmen and their Successors', *Scottish Studies*, vol. 13, Edinburgh, 1969.

MacAlister, E. F. B., *Sir Donald MacAlister of Tarbert*, London, 1935.

Mackay, F. F., *MacNeill of Carskey: His Estate Journal 1703–1743*, Edinburgh, 1955.

Sage, Revd. Donald, *Memorabilia Domestica: or Parish Life in the North of Scotland*, 2nd edn, William Rae, Wick, and John Menzies, Edinburgh, 1899.

8 'As Long As Grass Grows'

Birsay Report, *General Medical Services in the Highlands and Islands*. Cmnd 3257.

Bumsted, J. M., *The People's Clearance, 1770–1815*, Edinburgh University Press, 1982.

Cooper, Derek, *Road to the Isles: Travellers in the Hebrides 1770–1914*, Richard Drew, Glasgow, 1990.

Cullen, L. M., & Smout, T. C., *Comparative Aspects of Scottish & Irish Economic & Social History 1600–1900*, Edinburgh, 1977.

Day, J. P., *Public Administration in the Highlands and Islands of Scotland*, London, 1918.

Dewar Report, *Report of the Committee on the Highlands and Islands Medical Services*, HMSO (Cmnd 6559), 1912.

Grigor, Iain Fraser, *Mightier Than A Lord: The Highland Crofters Struggle for the Land*, Acair, Stornoway, 1979.

Grimble, Ian, *The Trial of Patrick Sellar: The Tragedy of the Highland Evictions*, Routledge & Kegan Paul, London, 1962.

Hunter, J., *The Making of the Crofting Community*, Edinburgh, 1976.

Mackenzie, Alexander, *History of the Highland Clearances*, Melven Press, Perth, 1979.

Maclean, Malcolm, & Carrell, Christopher, (eds), *As an Fhearann: From the Land*, Mainstream, Edinburgh, An Lanntair, Stornoway, & Third Eye Centre, Glasgow, 1986. In Gaelic and English, a splendidly illustrated book of essays by leading writers on Highland history, people and land. The canny reproduction of twee and facetious tourist postcards alongside photographs of real Highland life and the interpretations of inspired modern art, set the Gaels and their history in a proper perspective.

MacNeill, R., 'Remarks on the public health of the insular rural districts of Scotland', *Edinburgh Medical Journal*, vol. xxxiii, 25, 1887–8

Mitchell, G. A. G., 'Anatomical and resurrectionist activities in northern Scotland' in *Journal of the History of Medicine*, 4, 417–430.

Parman, S. 'Curing beliefs and practices in the Outer Hebrides' *Folklore*, vol. 88, 1977, 107–109.

Richards, Eric, *The Leviathan of Wealth*, London, 1973.

– 'Patterns of Highland Discontent, 1790–1860', in R. Quinault and J. Stevenson, (eds), *Popular Protest and Public Order: Six Studies in British History 1790–1920*, London, 1974.

– *A History of the Highland Clearances*, vol. 1: *Agrarian Transformation and the Evictions 1746–1886*, London, 1982; vol. 2: *Emigration, Protests, Reasons*, London, 1985.

Royal College of Physicians of Edinburgh, *Statement regarding the Existing Deficiency of Medical Practitioners in the Highlands and Islands*, Edinburgh, 1852.

Scottish Record Office, *Conditions in Highlands & Islands*, HH 65.

Smith, R., 'Consumption in the Highlands and Islands to the West of Scotland' and 'On the cause of phthisis in the Hebrides and West Highlands', *Edinburgh Medical Journal*, vol. xxviii, Edinburgh, 1872–3.

Stewart of Garth, David, *Sketches of the Character, Manners, and Present State of the Highlanders of Scotland*, 2 vols., Edinburgh, 1822. Reprinted, John Donald, 1977.

Temperley, Alan, *Tales of the North Coast*, Research Publishing Company, London, 1977.

9   A Future for the Past?

Griggs, Barbara, Green Pharmacy: A History of Herbal Medicine, Norman & Hobhouse, 1981.

Vogel, Virgil, *American Indian Medicine*, University of Oklahoma, 1970.

World Health, June, 1983. This entire issue of the World Health Organisation's official illustrated magazine is devoted to modern medicine's uses for traditional healing and the possibilities for the future.

II MATERIA MEDICA

GENERAL

Carmichael, A., *Carmina Gadelica*, 6 vols. Edinburgh, 1900–71; and in an English-only version, Floris Books, Edinburgh, 1992.

Macdonald, Revd. Norman, 'Notes on Gaelic Folklore II', *Arv: Tidskrift för Nordisk Folkminnesforskring: Journal of Scandinavian Folklore*, vol. 17, Uppsala & Copenhagen 1961.

McNeill, F. M., *The Silver Bough*, vol. 1, MacLellan, Glasgow, 1957.

Pennant, Thomas, *A Tour in Scotland and Voyage to the Hebrides*, Chester, 1772.

Shaw, M. F., *Folksongs and Folklore of South Uist*, Routledge & Kegan Paul, London, 1955.

Martindale's Extra Pharmacopoeia, Royal Pharmaceutical Society, London, is updated every few years. The first edition was published in 1883 and the most recent in 1993.

10 Waters, Wells and Healing Springs

Banks, Mary Macleod, *British Calendar Customs: Scotland*, vol. I, Folklore Society, London, 1937. Healing wells feature on 125–70.

Barrett, Dom Michael, *A Calendar of Scottish Saints*, Fort Augustus, 1919.

Bord, Colin and Janet, *Sacred Waters: Holy Wells and Water Lore in Britain and Ireland*, Granada, London, 1985.

MacKinlay, J.M., *The Folklore of Scottish Lochs and Streams*, William Hodge, Glasgow 1893. Reprinted, Llanerch, 1993.

Manson, D., *On the Strathpeffer Spa*, Inverness, 1866.

Morris, Ruth and Frank, *Scottish Healing Wells: healing, holy, wishing and fairy wells of the mainland of Scotland*, Alethea Press, Sandy, Bedfordshire, 1982.

Nicolaisen, W. F. H., *Scottish Place-names*, Batsford, London, 1976.

Thompson, T., 'On the Mineral Waters of Scotland', *Glasgow Medical Journal*, vol. 1, 20, Glasgow, 1828.

Watson, W. J., *History of the Celtic Place-names of Scotland*, Edinburgh & London, 1926; reprinted, Irish Academic Press, Dublin, 1986.

11 The Enchantment of Stone and Metal

Davidson, Thomas, 'Animal Treatment in Eighteenth-Century Scotland', *Scottish Studies*, vol. 4.

Black, George F, 'Scottish Charms and Amulets', *PSAS*, vol. 27, 1892–3, 433–526.

12 Of Mice, Horns, and Butterflies

Forbes, Alexander, *Gaelic Names of Beasts (Mammalia), Birds, Fishes, Insects, Reptiles, etc.*, Oliver & Boyd, Edinburgh, 1905.

Mackenzie, Donald A., 'Oriental Elements in Scottish Mythology', *TGSI*, vol.31, 1922–24, 116–132.

13 Rituals, Charms and Incantations

Campbell, John Gregorson, *Witchcraft and Second Sight in the Highlands & Islands of Scotland*, MacLehose, Glasgow, 1902.

MacBain, A., 'Gaelic Incantations', *TGSI*, vol. 17, 1894.

Macdonald, Alexander, 'Medical Spells and Charms of the Highlands', *Celtic Magazine* 13, 1887–8, 34–40.

—*Story and Song from Loch Ness-side*, Northern Counties Newspapers, Inverness, 1914, especially 175–83.

Mackenzie, William, 'Gaelic Incantations, Charms and Blessings of the Hebrides', in *TGSI* vol. 18, 1891–2, 97–182.

Meek, Donald, (ed.), *The Campbell Collection of Gaelic Proverbs and Proverbial Sayings*, collected by the Revd. Duncan M. Campbell, Gaelic Society of Inverness, 1978.

14 Herbal

Cameron, John, *Gaelic Names of Plants*, Blackwood, Edinburgh & London, 2nd rev. edn, 1900.

Fairweather, Barbara, *Highland Plant Lore*, Glencoe & North Lorn Folk Museum, undated. Repr. in Fairweather's *Highland Heritage*, Glencoe & North Lorn Folk Museum, 1984, 87–100.

Forsyth, A. A., *British Poisonous Plants*, Bulletin 161, Ministry of Agriculture, Fisheries & Food, HMSO, London, 1976. A handy reminder of the varying powers of nature to those who would have it that all plants – except for a few notoriously toxic ones – are benign in influence; and it also enhances respect for the folk healers' knowledge.

Grieve, M., *A Modern Herbal*, Jonathan Cape, London, 1931.

Grigson, Geoffrey, *The Englishman's Flora*, Phoenix, London, 1958. Despite its title this delightful and informative book contains a considerable amount of folklore material from Scottish, Irish and Welsh sources.

Hogan, F. E., *Luibhleabhrán: Irish & Scottish Gaelic Names of Plants*, 1900.

Le Strange, Richard, *A History of Herbal Plants*, Angus & Robertson, London, 1977.

Levy, Juliette de Baïracli, *The Illustrated Herbal Handbook*, 2nd rev. edn, Faber & Faber, London, 1982.

Lightfoot, John, *Flora Scotica*, 2 vols., London, 1777.

MacFarlane, Angus, 'Gaelic Names of Plants: Study of their Uses and Lore', in *TGSI*, vol. 32, 1924–5, 1–48.

McNeill, Malcolm, *Colonsay*, 1910.

Surey-Gent, Sonia, & Morris, Gordon, *Seaweed: A User's Guide*, Whittet Books, London, 1987.

Vickery, Roy, (ed.), *Plant Lore Studies*, Folklore Society, Mistletoe Series, vol. 18, 1984.

HEALING THREADS:
INDEXES

Gaelic (Index B) and botanical (C) names of herbs given in chapter 14 follow the main index. A further English index (D) gives plants, spices, etc, where they appear other than in alphabetical order in chapter 14. Routine materials such as butter are not itemised, neither are *forms (e.g.* poultices) of preparations which occur frequently. Words in bold type are to related references.

Aberdeenshire, 178
abortion, 18, 96
abscesses, 211; **quinsy, teeth**
Achadh na h-Annaide, 130
Achmore, 163
Achnashellach, 87
Adomnán, 37–8, 129, 155, 158
Aengus Céile Dé, Litany of, 249
Africa, 4–6
age, ageing, 18, 55, 64, 68, 69,
    78, 88, 89, 96, 116, 136, 139,
    141, 149, 155, 157, 216, 223
agriculture, 19, 32, 108, 114,
    118, 123
ague, 233; **fevers**
Aird nan Laogh, 68
Airmedh, 30, 31
alchemy, 56
alcohol, 32, 115–6, 122, 205,
    249; advice on, 59–60, 115,
    131; ale & beer, 115–6, 159,
    184, 206–7, 210, 212, 224;
    heather ale, 116, 216, 222,
    249; brewing/distilling, 16,
    32, 115–6, 193, 209–10, 236,
    249; drunkenness, 115, 205,
    249; hangover, 205; methylated

spirit, 163; rum, 116; whisky,
    59–60, 98–99, 115–6, 171,
    174, 181, 206, 211, 229, 245;
    wine, 59–60, 88, 99, 181, 215,
    217, 219; ritual use, 98–9, 217
Alexander I, 46
Alexander Severus, 30
America, 70, 162, 186, 208; native
    medicine, 24, 136
anaemia, 132
anaesthetic, 16, 236
Anaxagoras, 62
angels, 37, 41, 153, 166
Anglesey, 29
Anglo-Saxon leechbooks, 196
Angus (place), 34, 45, 152
Angus Og, Lord of the Isles, 45
annats, 130–131
aphorisms, 55–6
aphrodisiacs, see **love potions**
Apollo, Romano-Celtic, 91, 178
apoplexy, see **stroke**
apothecaries, 8, 14, 70, 78
appendicitis, 160
appetisers, 88, 211, 212, 213,
    229–30, 243
Applecross, 87, 138

Index

Index

Index

Index

Index

Index

INDEX C -Botanical names of plants in chapter 14

Index

INDEX D -English names of plants
Note: The plants, trees, etc, given
in bold type also have alphabetically
ordered entries in chapter 14 which are
not given here; where plants occur *out
of sequence* in that chapter they are given
below. Highly processed materials such
as camphor (from a type of cinnamon),
Persian gum (from acacia) and opium
are in the main index.